ALLERGIES AND INFECTIOUS DISEASES

ALLERGIES AND INFECTIOUS DISEASES

ALLERGIES AND AUTISM
Michael J. Dochniak and Denise H. Dunn
2010. ISBN: 978-1-60876-352-8

ALLERGIES AND INFECTIOUS DISEASES

ALLERGIES AND AUTISM

MICHAEL J. DOCHNIAK
AND
DENISE H. DUNN

Nova Science Publishers, Inc.
New York

For permission to use material from this book please contact us:
Telephone 631-231-7269; Fax 631-231-8175
Web Site: http://www.novapublishers.com

NOTICE TO THE READER

The Publisher has taken reasonable care in the preparation of this book, but makes no expressed or implied warranty of any kind and assumes no responsibility for any errors or omissions. No liability is assumed for incidental or consequential damages in connection with or arising out of information contained in this book. The Publisher shall not be liable for any special, consequential, or exemplary damages resulting, in whole or in part, from the readers' use of, or reliance upon, this material.

Independent verification should be sought for any data, advice or recommendations contained in this book. In addition, no responsibility is assumed by the publisher for any injury and/or damage to persons or property arising from any methods, products, instructions, ideas or otherwise contained in this publication.

This publication is designed to provide accurate and authoritative information with regard to the subject matter covered herein. It is sold with the clear understanding that the Publisher is not engaged in rendering legal or any other professional services. If legal or any other expert assistance is required, the services of a competent person should be sought. FROM A DECLARATION OF PARTICIPANTS JOINTLY ADOPTED BY A COMMITTEE OF THE AMERICAN BAR ASSOCIATION AND A COMMITTEE OF PUBLISHERS.

LIBRARY OF CONGRESS CATALOGING-IN-PUBLICATION DATA

Dochniak, Michael J.
  Allergies and autism / authors, Michael J. Dochniak, Denise H. Dunn.
      p. ; cm.
  Includes bibliographical references and index.
  ISBN 978-1-60876-352-8 (softcover)
  1. Autism--Immunological aspects. 2. Latex allergy. I. Dunn, Denise H. II. Title.
  [DNLM: 1. Autistic Disorder--etiology. 2. Hypersensitivity, Immediate--complications. 3. Latex--immunology. 4. Latex Hypersensitivity--complications. WM 203.5 D637a 2009]
  RC553.A88D63 2009
  616.85'882071--dc22
                                                                                    2009035680

Published by Nova Science Publishers, Inc. ✛ *New York*

CONTENTS

PREFACE

The immune-response perspective in cognitive development is intended to explore how certain environmental proteins and genetic factors affect neuro-cognitive development and mental health thereafter. Specifically, naturally occurring proteins are known to cause severe and pervasive immune responses. More specifically, environmental antigenic/allergenic proteins may trigger IgE mediated reaction antibodies that influence cross-react immune responses to homologous exogenous/endogenous proteins. Repeated exposure to antigenic/allergenic proteins has been shown to cause an increased incidence of sensitization, adverse allergic reactions, and even death through anaphylactic shock.

ACKNOWLEDGMENTS

Dr. Michael Keenan, teachers are silently inclusive in the questions we ask and the answers we seek.

James Judson, Chief Executive Officer and President of Jasmine Elastomeric; in the most professional manner you deal with the yin and yang of *Hevea brasiliensis* natural-latex.

American Chemical, a thoughtful company with people that care.

Artists/Illustrators: Daniel D. Hennes; Basil S. Dochniak; Duane J. Hennes, Katie Flint and Nicole Mizoguchi.

ABOUT THE AUTHORS

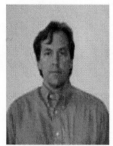

Michael John Dochniak is a researcher in the field of *Hevea brasiliensis* natural-latex induced Autism. Michael has been a noted writer, speaker, researcher, and inventor in chemistry for more than 20 years and is the author of a paper entitled, *Autism Spectrum Disorders-Exogenous Protein Insult* for the journal Medical Hypotheses.

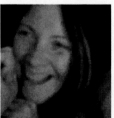

Denise Harmony Dunn is an early childhood educator in Minnesota. Harmony works closely with families, infants, autistic children and adults. She has been teaching for more than 15 years, is researching how environmental protein-insult affects the etiology of disease, and has co-authored a chapter entitled, *Antigenic/Allergenic Rubber Proteins and Environmental Regulation* for Nova Scientific Publishers.

INTRODUCTION

Allergy induced Autism explores how certain proteins induce hyper adaptive-immunity affecting Autism Spectrum Disorders. Environmental proteins can cause immune responses that are severe, pervasive, and perpetuating. Specifically, *Hevea brasiliensis* natural rubber latex (natural-latex) contains many antigenic proteins that are considered potentially harmful allergens. Repeated exposure to such allergens has been shown to cause frequent immune responses affecting the occurrence and longevity of allergies in atopic children. Natural-latex has seen a dramatic increase in usage over the last thirty years particularly in the health care industry and it is often used in the manufacture of infant products including baby bottle nipples, pacifiers, and toys. Repeated exposure to the natural-latex allergens has been shown to perpetuate other immune responses including food allergies based on antibody miscommunication or cross-reactivity. Adding clarity to the etiology of Autism Spectrum Disorders, allergies increase the expression of neurotrophin including neuron growth factor. It is known that neuron growth factor dramatically affects neural growth and synaptic pruning. Allergy sensitive children are more susceptible to atypical neurological development. Within the Autism Spectrum, some allergy sensitive individuals have exceptional cognitive skills in mathematics, music, scientific creativity, and writing while other allergy sensitive individuals have severe and pervasive impairment in thinking, feeling, language, and sociability. It will be shown that the timing, frequency, intensity, and type of exposure to the allergens in natural-latex can induce hyper-adaptive immunity; effecting the incidence and degree of atypicality of autistic behaviors. Adaptive immunity gives medical science new insight into brain development, many individuals on the Autism Spectrum have shown that the intellectual progression/regression of mankind rests on the shoulders of immunity.

Dain is a person with Regressive Autism and his allergy induced Autism experience is described in this book.

Chapter I

ALLERGY INDUCED AUTISM

Autism is an extremely variable disorder. – Temple Grandin

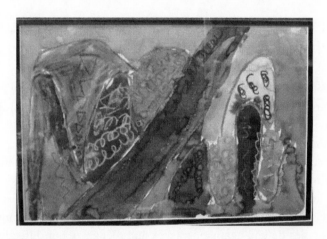

A time of anticipated celebration, a time of joy as brightly colored party balloons, wrapped gifts, paper plates, and inscribed napkins decorated picnic tables for family and friends gathered to share vanilla-frosted cake at Dain's 2nd birthday. Dain playfully mouthed an inflated natural-latex balloon while others cheerfully watched and sang happy birthday. Within the balloon was an invasive danger that would soon severely threaten and change his life forever. Shortly after playing with the balloon, Dain's health steadily regressed as his adaptive immune system recognized and attacked the natural-latex proteins that had transferred, through inhalation and dermal absorption, from the balloon and into his body. As the allergic response progressed and intensified his health worsened, frightened parents comforted their child as each labored breath failed to change the dark-purple color in his lips from oxygen starved blood. Rushed to the hospital emergency room, a nurse quickly injected adrenaline into his tiny shoulder. A mask supplied a steady stream of oxygen and intravenous tubes dripped essential fluids into his arm, rapidly turning his lips a safe pink color again allowing this atopic child to overcome a severe allergic reaction and live another day. Before leaving the hospital, a Doctor discussed his allergy situation. It was recommended that a nebulizer be used at home to relieve any recurrent asthmatic symptoms. The treatments helped his breathing but failed to address its underlying cause and progression - his adaptive immune system was hyper-active and out of control. Within a year, Dain would experience many more allergic manifestations and be diagnosed with Regressive Autism; thereafter helplessly locked *forever* in a world of behavioral atypicality.

ARE NATURAL-LATEX ALLERGIES PERPETUATED BY THE HARMLESS ASPECT OF THE FAMILIAR?

The Webster II Dictionary defines an allergy as a hypersensitive reaction to a substance harmless to most people. But for many people, it is well documented that allergies can be severely debilitating and even deadly.

The immune system comprises some of the most expressive, adaptive, and complicated chemistry in the human body. There are primarily two types of immunity; innate immunity and adaptive immunity. In innate immunity, antibodies like immunoglobulin-G and immunoglobulin-M protect us from being destroyed by infectious microorganisms. In adaptive immunity, immunoglobulin-E (IgE) antibodies defend against parasites and recognize non-infectious proteins called antigens causing allergies. IgE antibodies are adaptive and can cross-react with other beneficial proteins including food proteins. This cross-react miscommunication is influenced by many factors including protein homology, antibody expression, androgen expression, comorbidity, genetics, and epigenetics. Everyone has the potential to acquire allergies and it is this immunity that affects the development of Autism Spectrum Disorders.

Are Childrens Immune systems more sensitive to Allergens Compared to Adults?

A study has shown that the levels of IgE antibody blood markers for allergies were significantly higher in children compared to their parents. On average, the levels of IgE antibodies in children were three times higher than their parents [1]. The Environmental Protection Agency recognizes that children are more susceptible to chemicals than adults. As an example, within the *Children's Environmental Health Center* website it states, "For many reasons, children are likely to be more vulnerable than adults to the effects of environmental contaminants. To better understand the effects of these exposures on children's health, the *Centers for Children's Environmental Health and Disease Prevention Research* was established to explore ways to reduce children's health risks from environmental factors" [2].

Why have Childhood Allergies become more Prevalent?

Allergen exposure has caused a dramatic increase in childhood allergies. Specifically, allergens that have dramatically increased over the last thirty years are the proteins from natural-latex. Natural-latex is extracted from the Para rubber tree and is suspected to contain at least sixty different allergenic proteins. (Note; in the following chapters, the term natural-latex will be used exclusively to describe *Hevea brasiliensis* natural rubber latex) Repeated exposure to these allergens has been shown to cause an increased incidence of sensitization, adverse allergic reactions, and even death through anaphylactic shock. Furthermore, natural-latex allergens can act as a catalyst for the development of other allergic manifestations including food allergies.

Natural-latex allergy is associated with adaptive immunity and immunoglobulin-E (IgE) antibodies. Compared to other antibodies free-floating in the blood stream, IgE antibodies have low concentration (approximately one-thousandth of a percent) and a short half-life (approximately two days). IgE antibodies are specific to a select group of antigen, rather than a wide range, and are extremely biologically active despite low concentrations in circulation. This is because IgE antibodies bind to high-affinity receptors on the surface of mast cells and basophils, so that these cells may be highly sensitive to antigens even when the concentration of IgE antibodies in the circulation is very low. Thus, unlike other immunoglobulin antibodies, IgE antibodies play a major role in reactivity to an allergen. IgE antibody expression and selectivity may play a critical role in the onset of allergy induced Autism. For example, an immune response associated with the allergens in natural-latex may induce lymphocytes like plasma B-cells and memory B-cells to form IgE antibodies that target homologous proteins (i.e., cross-react). Several examples of cross-react immune responses to homologous exogenous-proteins and homologous endogenous-proteins will be described in chapters 3, 4, and 5.

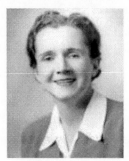

Rachel Carson

In the book entitled *Silent Spring* wildlife biologist Rachel Carson taught that man-made chemicals like pesticides and insecticides that become universally common or repetitive can assume "the harmless aspect of the familiar" [3]. In parallel the allergens in natural-latex, some of which are suspected to be natural insecticides, have attained *the harmless aspect of the familiar*. Even though many of the health and safety hazards of natural-latex are well understood, exploitation and a comfortable dependence on such a material continues to stress children's health based on an inertia sustained by *the harmless aspect of the familiar*.

Repeated exposure to the allergens in natural-latex often increases the specific-antibody population affecting the intensity and duration of the immune response. Alternatively, exclusion of the allergenic proteins inhibits re-activation of associated T-cells and B-cells allowing such cells to substantially decay, dampening the immune response. Therefore, it is now understood in medical science that the best means to eliminate the incidence and prevalence of natural-latex allergy is avoidance. All products that come into contact with individuals having a developing nervous system should be reviewed for natural-latex in that the critical period for the development of the brain is from about three weeks to about sixteen weeks, although major structures of the brain continue to develop throughout childhood.

Science and industry has clearly shown that the allergens in natural-latex can be harmful. Both continue to deal with the absolute that exposure can cause severe allergic reactions in atopic children. Most recently, exclusionary measures have been initiated in hospitals and forward thinking companies have developed effective protein extraction methods in an effort to provide Ultra-low protein natural-latex.

Over the last sixty years science has failed to discover the cause of Autism Spectrum Disorders. Although defined behaviorally, it is becoming clearer that it is immunologically based. The complexity and variability of allergy induced Autism has made a definitive etiology elusive in that science demands consistency and repeatability. Interacting variables including the static nature of adaptive immunity, genetic susceptibility, epigenetics, androgen expression, endogenous protein expression, and many other co-morbid factors has contributed to it complexity. One thing is certain, when the adaptive immune system is genetically susceptible to atopy and continuously stressed, brain development is altered.

Despite the lack of prevalence data on Autism Spectrum Disorders worldwide, there are emerging trend numbers that suggest that tens of millions of children and adults have Autism Spectrum Disorders. As the numbers increase, the resulting costs of this lifelong condition on national economies rise concurrently. It is estimated that by 2010, the cost of caring for the estimated 1.75 million Americans with Autism Spectrum Disorders will reach $90 billion per year. In countries such as India, Russia and Nigeria, these costs could cripple a nation's health and education budgets within a few years. While the World Health Organization does not maintain global statistics on the prevalence of Autism Spectrum Disorders, its 2007 Global Burden of Disease report on mental and neurological disorders highlighted the critical situation the world faces with a growing population that includes those with Autism [4].

In the following chapters, biological models and theoretical models are used to explain how the allergens in natural-latex can induce cross-reactivity and trigger hyper adaptive-immunity, affecting atypical neuro-cognitive development in children.

REFERENCES

[1] Brian Reid (2005). Levels of Blood Marker for Allergies Higher in Children than Parents, Suggesting Real Rise in Allergy Rates: Presented at AAP. http://www.docguide.com/news/content.nsf/news/8525697700573E188525 70980050B3D6.

[2] Children's Environmental Health Centers. EPA Website, http://es.epa.gov/ ncer/childrenscenters/index.html

[3] Rachel Carson. (1962) Silent Spring, Houghton Mifflin Publishers.

[4] Autism Society of America. Incidence numbers from other countries. http://www.autism-society.org/site/PageServer?pagename=community_world_incidence

Chapter II

AUTISM SPECTRUM DISORDERS

I didn't get where I am today by not being autistic. -Larry Arnold
Those who make a difference are those who are different. – Harmony Dunn

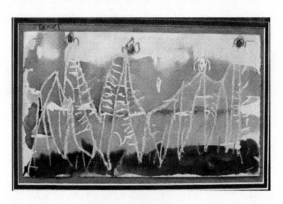

As Dain's allergy induced Autism progressed, more atypical behaviors crept into his life. Sitting on top of the refrigerator opening and closing the freezer door is one such behavior. The combined visual sensation of height, depth, and a thrill of opening and closing the door was his self-initiated experiment. Both parents submitted and allowed this to continue based on the realization that forced exclusion would just initiate him to seek an alternative atypical behavior. "How can this be happening?" is often a recurrent thought for parents' and professionals when dealing with severely mentally-disabled children whose Autism Spectrum Disorder diagnosis is 'Not Otherwise Specified'

DOES THE INTELLECTUAL PROGRESSION OF MANKIND REST ON THE SHOULDERS OF IMMUNITY?

Many on the Autism Spectrum have severe and pervasive impairment in thinking, feeling, language, and sociability. Hyper adaptive-immunity and subsequent atypical neural development (e.g., neural over-connectivity) may over-facilitate the amplification of certain types of perceptions and focus adversely affecting behavior. Alternatively, some on the Autism Spectrum have exceptional cognitive skills in mathematics, music, scientific creativity, and writing. In these individuals, hyper adaptive-immunity and subsequent neural over-connectivity may facilitate the amplification of certain types of perceptions and focus beyond the level achieved by immuno-typical individuals.

Scientists now understand that the differential onset of early Classical Autism and Regressive Autism indicates an etiology influenced by many factors including immunology, environmental insult, genetics, and epigenetics. Historically, one of the early theories on the cause of Autism Spectrum Disorders was referred to as "refrigerator mother". The term *refrigerator mother* was coined around the year 1950 as a label for mothers of children diagnosed with Autism. These mothers were often blamed for their children's atypical behaviors which included rigid rituals, speech difficulty, and self-isolation. As a result, many mothers of children on the autistic spectrum suffered from blame, guilt, and self-doubt.

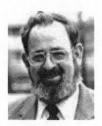

Bernard Rimland

In 1964, the psychologist Bernard Rimland published a book that signaled the emergence of a counter-explanation to the established misconceptions about the causes of Autism. His book, *Infantile Autism: the Syndrome and its Implications for a Neural Theory of Behavior*, attacked the 'refrigerator mother' hypothesis directly. Bernard Rimland's efforts have influenced a modern day consensus on the cause of Autism Spectrum Disorders, a combination of environmental insult and genetic susceptibility.

Autism Spectrum Disorders are often first diagnosed in early childhood and range from a severe form called Autistic Disorder Not Otherwise Specified to a much milder form called Asperger Syndrome. This syndrome was named after Austrian pediatrician Hans Asperger who, in 1944, described children in his practice who lacked verbal communication skills, demonstrated limited empathy with their peers, and were physically clumsy. It is generally understood that there is no single treatment for Asperger Syndrome, and the effectiveness of particular interventions is supported by only limited data. Intervention is aimed at improving symptoms and function. The principle support of management is behavioral therapy, focusing on specific deficits to address poor communication skills, obsessive or repetitive routines, and physical clumsiness. It is suggested that most individuals with Asperger syndrome can cope with their difference, but many continue to need support and encouragement to maintain a healthy and independent lifestyle.

From a humanistic viewpoint, some have advocated a shift in attitudes toward the view that Asperger Syndrome is a difference, rather than a disability. Others say that Autism is another way of thinking and being. There are individuals on the Autism Spectrum who are very comfortable with their difference. As an example, the quote used in the beginning of this chapter is from an autistic man who said, "I didn't get where I am today by not being autistic." Alternatively, there are individuals on the Autism Spectrum who are less comfortable about their difference. A teenage boy diagnosed with Asperger Syndrome was asked if he liked being called autistic and he said, "Calling me autistic is hard because of how people treat me".

Are Autism Spectrum Disorders Increasing?

A paper published in the American Psychological Society titled, *three reasons not to believe in an Autism epidemic* describes why some laypersons mistakenly believe that there is an Autism epidemic. The authors suggest that people are unaware of the purposeful broadening of diagnostic criteria, coupled with deliberately greater public awareness; they accept the unwarranted conclusions of the Medical Investigation of Neuro-developmental Disorders Institute study; and they fail to realize that Autism was not even an *Individual with Disabilities Education Act* reporting category until the early 1900s. It is also suggested that incremental increases will most likely continue until the schools are identifying and serving the number of children identified in epidemiological studies. Furthermore, apart from a desire to be aligned with scientific reasoning, there are other reasons not to believe in an Autism epidemic. Epidemics solicit causes; false epidemics solicit false causes. What message do we send autistic children and adults when we call their increasing number an epidemic, a pandemic, or a scourge? Increasing Autism rates are most likely due to non-catastrophic mechanisms, such as purposely broader diagnostic criteria and greater public awareness [1].

Research indicates that the incidence of Autism Spectrum Disorders is rising. As an example, For example, a study indicates that most recently there has been an epidemic of developmental, learning, and behavioral disabilities in children. The study showed that the apparent rise in numbers is not the result of "Diagnosis Shifting" and that Autism is increasing with successively younger children, particularly those born between 1987 and 1992 [2].

The United States government is becoming more sensitive to the issue that Autism rates are increasing. In 2007 Congress passed a resolution designating April 2007 as "National Autism Awareness Month". The resolution supported efforts to increase research funding into the causes and treatment of Autism, improve training, and support individuals with Autism and those who care for individuals with Autism.

The resolution was written as follows:

Whereas designating April 2007 as `National Autism Awareness Month' will increase public awareness of the need to support individuals with Autism and the family members and medical professionals who care for individuals with Autism:

Now, therefore, be it Resolved, That the Senate—

(i) Designates April 2007 as 'National Autism Awareness Month';

(ii) Recognizes and commends the parents and relatives of children with Autism for their sacrifice and dedication in providing for the special needs of children with Autism and for absorbing significant financial costs for specialized education and support services;

(iii) Supports the goal of increasing Federal funding for aggressive research to learn the root causes of Autism, identify the best methods of early intervention and treatment, expand programs for individuals with Autism across their lifespan, and promote understanding of the special needs of people with Autism;

(iv) Stresses the need to begin early intervention services soon after a child has been diagnosed with Autism, noting that early intervention strategies are the primary therapeutic options for young people with Autism, and that early intervention significantly improves the outcome for people with Autism and can reduce the level of funding and services needed to treat people with Autism later in life;

(x) Supports the Federal Government's more than 30-year-old commitment to provide States with 40 percent of the costs needed to educate children with disabilities under part B of the Individuals with Disabilities Education Act 20 U.S.C. 1411 et seq.;

(xi) Recognizes the shortage of appropriately trained teachers who have the skills and support necessary to teach, assist, and respond to special needs students, including those with Autism, in our school systems; and

(xii) Recognizes the importance of worker training programs that are tailored to the needs of developmentally disabled persons, including those with Autism, and notes that people with Autism can be, and are, productive members of the workforce if they are given appropriate support, training, and early intervention services. [3]

It is clear that the Autism epidemic is real. An etiology must be able too explain the extreme range of cognitive atypicality within the Autism Spectrum including severe mental retardation to brilliance. Hyper adaptive-immunity associated with allergy induced Autism is an etiology that may provide such an explanation for a subgroup of individuals on the Autism Spectrum.

What is the Evolution of Autism Spectrum Disorders?

Two pioneering models of evolutionary theory, Darwinian/Wallace selection and Mendelian genetics, have failed to shed light on the cause of Autism Spectrum Disorders. Charles Darwin conceded that natural selection is not the sole mechanism of evolutionary change and Alfred Wallace asserted that natural selection could not account for the human brain. Furthermore, Gregory Mendel's genetic models of evolution and modern genetic-research techniques have failed to decipher the genetic code(s) in that a Mendelian (single-gene) mutation or a single chromosome abnormality has not been discovered. Adaptive immunity may be a model that can be used to shed light on the evolution of Autism Spectrum Disorders; the atypical expression of biochemicals after immune responses has been shown to affect neurological development.

Do Allergies Affect human Intelligence?

Mammals are the only organisms that produce IgE antibodies. In humans, the expression and activity of such antibodies may play an important role in brain development in that allergies induce the over-expression of neurotrophin. The over-expression of neurotrophin and its affect on neurological development will be discussed in Chapter 4.

Genetic research has shown us that our closest relative is the chimpanzee. It may be understood that humans are intellectually different than the Chimpanzee because of immunity. A study indicates that humans and chimpanzees have remarkably dissimilar adaptive immunity. For example, research at the University of California – San Diego has shown that human T-cells, which are an important orchestrator of the immune system, respond much more robustly than chimpanzee cells do [4].

The recent proliferation of Autism Spectrum Disorders has presented clues to the evolution of the human brain and allergies play a critical role. It may be understood that the antithesis of "survival of the fittest" is mankind. Cognitive atypicality in the Autism Spectrum, ranging from severe mental retardation to fragile genius, based on stressed adaptive-immunity may be one of the most significant evolutionary processes of our species.

REFERENCES

[1] Morton Ann Gernsbacher, Michelle Dawson, H. Hill Goldsmith. (2005). Three Reasons Not to Believe in an Autism Epidemic. *American Psychological Society, Volume 14*, Number 2, pages 55-58.

[2] NAAR funded Research Leads New Study. (2005). Examining Autism Prevalence. http://www.autismspeaks.org/inthenews/naar_archive/examining_autism_pr evalence.php.

[3] govtrack.us. (2007). National Autism Awareness Month. http://www. govtrack.us/congress/bill.xpd?bill=sr110-78.

[4] Bio-Medicine. (2006). T cell 'brakes' lost during human evolution. http://news.bio-medicine.org/medicine-news-3/T-cell-brakes-lost-during-human-evolution-5003-1/

Chapter III

ALLERGENS

Where is the wisdom we have lost in knowledge? – T.S. Eliot

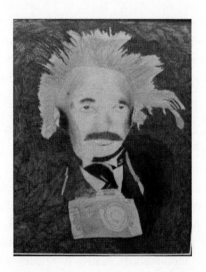

Dain's susceptibility to allergies was evident at a very young age. Frequent rashes, asthma, constant runny nose, and sneezing were a few signs that his adaptive immune system was hyper-active. Unwilling to regularly eat solid food and a stubborn refusal to drink from a cup, he was often fed bottles of milk using natural-latex nipples. His lips were often very red and swollen after eating. Ignorance on the hazards of natural-latex, and repeated exposure, likely caused and/or intensified Dain's allergies fueling his Regressive Autism.

WILL ULTRA LOW-PROTEIN NATURAL-LATEX BECOME ONE OF THE MOST IMPORTANT HEALTH AND SAFETY INITIATIVES OF THE 21ST CENTURY?

Before the first sea creature ventured from the ocean depths onto land, flora was firmly rooted in the soil. In this botanical realm, energy and nutrients absorbed from the sun, rain, and soil allowed plants and trees to transform carbon dioxide and other earthly elements into many complex chemicals including cellulose, carbohydrates, and proteins which strengthened its ability to adapt and survive. As an example, many of the proteins produce by the Para rubber tree (i.e., natural-latex) are considered defense proteins. These proteins can adversely affect our immune system and are considered chronic non-infectious agents or allergens.

Natural-latex allergies are the creation of nature and have likely stressed adaptive-immune systems far back in mankind's history. Exposure to rubber proteins by the exploitation of lacticiferous plants happened as early as 1600 B.C. Modern evidence has shown that the Mesoamericans, who had some of the most complex and advanced cultures including the Maya and the Aztec, used stabilized rubber from the plant Castilla elastica as early as 1600 B.C. Natural-latex as a protective material has a long history dating back to the 1800s. In the early 19th century, natural-latex became an important raw material in industrialized societies when Charles Goodyear discovered a chemical process (vulcanization) that cured the rubber to remove its "stickiness". Thereafter, natural-latex was transformed into a magnificent number of products. At present, it is estimated that more than 40,000 commercially available products are made with natural-latex.

The polyisoprene in natural-latex is a wonderful gift from nature. Its unique chemical and physical properties have made it a material of choice for many industrial and consumer applications. Studies have shown that natural-latex films have excellent strength and form an effective barrier to pathogens. These unique properties make it particularly useful in medical gloves and infant products including baby bottle nipples and pacifiers. Many other useful products formed from natural-latex include septums for medicinal vials, children toys, and food packaging.

Much of the natural rubber used today is from a milky white extract from the Hevea brasiliensis rubber tree. Hevea brasiliensis is mostly grown in Malaysia, Liberia, and Thailand as the crops flourishes in regions within 5 to 10 degrees of the equator and at moderate elevations. Tapping a rubber tree involves cutting channels into the bark (controlled wounding) and bleeding out the milky white extract. Natural-latex from Hevea brasiliensis is produced by special cells called laticifiers and is thought to be a defense against insect pathogens and possibly a site for the depositing of metabolic waste of the tree.

It is well known that the proteins in natural-latex may cause allergic reactions. For example, it is known that natural-latex contains about two to five percent protein by weight. Analytical tests indicate about two-hundred dissimilar proteins are present and about fifty to sixty are suspected allergens. The World Health Organization - International Union of Immunological Societies has assigned names to thirteen of these allergens designated *Hev-b* 1 through *Hev-b* 13. It is well known that exposure to these proteins can cause chronic disease and they are considered chronic non-infectious agents. Factors that affect immune sensitivity include repeated exposure through inhalation and/or dermal absorption and a genetic predisposition to atopy. The threshold of sensitivity to the allergens in natural-latex is unknown, although a significant number of highly atopic individuals remain hypersensitive to even minute quantities (parts per million).

The allergens in natural-latex that have been shown to significantly affect the level of immunoglobulin-E primed cells are the water soluble proteins (e.g., *Hev-b* 1-3). Health care workers have experienced an increased number of sensitization from the use of powdered gloves formed from natural-latex. The antigenic protein content of such gloves can vary greatly and is due in part to protein leaching processing techniques. The International Rubber Research and Development Board have suggested that the protein allergy problem appears to have been instigated by the appearance of some very poorly manufactured gloves and other natural-latex articles on the market. These were produced by entrepreneurs who were unaware of, or disregarded, normal natural-latex dipping plant management. At worst they failed to maintain cleanliness on their dipping lines thus permitting build ups of protein sediment in their dipping tanks. They also failed to ensure adequate leaching of their products, either through performing the operation too quickly, or through using contaminated water. This led to the marketing of some natural-latex products with very high protein levels. This in turn led to severe reactions in potentially sensitive individuals. There is also some evidence that the transfer of manufacture to natural rubber producing countries led to the use of fresh natural-latex, which contains higher levels, and may make the seasonal and clonal variations in protein levels more pronounced in the products manufactured from them [1].

The literature describes the natural-latex proteins' affinity for USP absorbable dusting powder and several papers have been presented on this subject confirming this interaction. The United States Food and Drug Administration have recognized this association and have recommended a limit on powder and extractable protein per glove. Allergen-laden glove powder is implicated as a major contributor to the widespread sensitization to natural-latex and associated workplace symptoms wherein the powder acts as a vector to spread the proteins [2].

Natural-latex is currently recognized as a hazardous material by the National Institute for Occupational Safety and Health. The following request was taken from the their website, "The National Institute for Occupational Safety and Health requests assistance in preventing allergic reactions to natural-latex among workers who use gloves and other products containing natural-latex. Natural-latex gloves have proved effective in preventing transmission of many infectious diseases to health care workers. But for some workers, exposures to natural-latex may result in skin rashes; hives; flushing; itching; nasal, eye, or sinus symptoms; asthma; and (rarely) shock. Reports of such allergic reactions to natural-latex have increased in recent years—especially among health care workers. At present, scientific data are incomplete regarding the natural history of natural-latex allergy. Also, improvements are needed in methods used to measure proteins causing natural-latex allergy. This alert presents the existing data and describes six case reports of workers who developed natural-latex allergy. The document also presents the Occupational Safety and Health organizations recommendations for minimizing natural-latex related health problems in workers while protecting them from infectious materials. These recommendations include reducing exposures, using appropriate work practices, training and educating workers, monitoring symptoms, and substituting non-natural-latex products when appropriate. The Occupational Safety and Health organization requests that employers, owners, editors of trade journals, safety and health officials, and labor unions bring the recommendations in this alert to the attention of all workers who may be exposed to natural-latex [3].

It has been estimated that approximately five percent of the population have an allergic sensitivity to the allergens in natural-latex. Furthermore, published data indicates that seventeen percent of American healthcare workers are sensitized to the natural-latex proteins [4].

Individuals can be exposed to natural-latex for many years and not experience sensitivity and then, without any known risk factor, become severely disabled with allergies. In the other extreme, individuals can experience a severe natural-latex allergy immediately after the first exposure. While studies repeatedly uncover high prevalence rates of natural-latex allergy, the nonspecific nature of symptoms often results in missed diagnosis in many sensitized persons. They then become at risk for progression to more serious allergic reactions.

A study that evaluated percutaneous penetration of natural-latex proteins concluded that the skin is not only a plausible route for sensitization but can be a major exposure route when the integument has been compromised [5].

Most recently, the adhesive industry has been responsive to the health and safety issues associated with natural-latex. For example, adhesive companies have developed hypoallergenic formulations, which are free of natural-latex, for medical-packaging applications. Although the price/performance relationship between natural-latex and synthetic rubber continues to give life to natural-latex based adhesives, research efforts continue to develop alternative water-based formulations that have an effective combination of properties including strong wet-tack and reduced dry-tack allowing them to compete with natural-latex adhesives. Surprisingly, natural-latex adhesives continue to be used in the packaging of Band-Aids [6].

In a follow-up study on natural-latex allergy in children, research showed that strict compliance with natural-latex avoidance instructions is essential both inside and outside the hospital and greater emphasis should be placed on reducing natural-latex exposure in the home and school environments in that such contact could maintain positive immunoglobulin-E antibody levels [7].

IgE antibody primed-cells that are programmed to target specific proteins can also bind to other structurally similar proteins (i.e., homologous) through a mechanism called cross-reaction. Biological models of homologous proteins that have been shown to cross-react with natural-latex include the following:

Wheat

In a study that evaluated the multi-domain protein wheat germ agglutinin, research compared the homologous amino acid sequences of Hevein and each of the four domains (A, B, C, and D) of wheat germ agglutinin and used them to construct a pseudo-phylogenetic tree relating these sequences to a hypothetical common ancestor sequence. In the crystal structure of the wheat germ agglutinin dimer, six pseudo-twofold rotational symmetry axes have previously been located in addition to the true twofold axis. Four of these relate two non-identical domains to each other in each of the four possible pairs constituting the sugar-binding sites (A1D2, A2D1, B1C2, and B2C1). The remaining two relate contiguous unique pairs of sugar-binding sites to each other (A1D2 to B1C2, and A2D1 to B2C1). These latter two sets of pairs are related to each other by the true twofold axis. Side chains that mediate sugar binding in the interfaces of each of the four pairs were found to be largely conserved. The sequence homology, taken together with these pseudo-symmetry elements in the dimer structure, suggests a pathway for the evolution of the four-domain molecule from a single-domain dimer that can be correlated with simultaneous development of the saccharide-binding sites [8].

There is no actual treatment for wheat allergies. A child with the allergies must avoid wheat and wheat-related products. This is one of the most difficult food allergies because wheat and wheat products are in so many things we eat. Anything containing flour, for instance, which includes many boxed, bottled and canned products, even frozen foods, would need to be avoided.

Pine Wood

Research has shown an immunoglobulin-E cross reaction between natural-latex and pine wood. A brief summary of the study is as follows: It is well known that Hevea brasiliensis natural-latex gloves can cause allergy among hospital personnel and that these Hevea brasiliensis natural-latex allergic persons develop cross reactions to fruits and vegetables. Little is known about cross reactions to other trees. In a patient with clinical allergy to Hevea brasiliensis natural-latex we found cross reacting immunoglobulin-E to components in a wood dust extract from Pine. The patient is a laboratory technician who had to stop working as technician because of allergic skin symptoms caused by using Hevea brasiliensis natural-latex gloves. Demonstration of Hevea brasiliensis natural-latex specific immunoglobulin-E in the patient serum was detected by Magic Lite (ALK-Abello) and immunoglobulin-E dot blots. Hevea brasiliensis natural-latex specific immunoglobulin-E was found to be class 3 in Magic Lite. In order to demonstrate cross reactions to other types of trees the following extracts were used: pine (Pinus Silvestris), beech (Fagus Sylvatica) and oak (Quercus Eurpaeus).These extracts were blotted on nitrocellulose and incubated with the patient serum. The dot blots showed that the serum contained immunoglobulin-E directed against the pine extract but not to beech and oak. Inhibition studies using Hevea brasiliensis natural-latex allergen coupled to magnetic beads showed inhibition of specific immunoglobulin-E against pine extract on dot blots. To the researchers' knowledge, this was the first report to demonstrate a cross reaction between Hevea brasiliensis natural-latex and pine wood [9].

Pine Rosin

Pine rosin can be a cross react allergen in individuals with Hevea brasiliensis natural-latex allergy. Swedish research has identified pine rosin in diapers. A brief description of their study is as follows: As part of the investigation of sources of exposure of rosin allergens, disposable diapers (napkins) common on the Swedish market were analyzed, using gas chromatography, to detect the main rosin compounds. Rosin components were detected in all diapers, the highest amounts in those from the 2 major producers. In these diapers, more rosin was found in the top layer, which is in close contact with the skin, than in the fluff. Despite the possibly minimal risk of induction of sensitization to rosin allergens in diapers, there is a real risk of elicitation of dermatitis in sensitive individuals, especially since penetration is enhanced by occlusion and irritation. Such material is not only used for infant diapers, but also for adult incontinence products and feminine hygiene products [10].

Euphorbiaceae Species

Research has shown that there is a cross reaction between Hevea brasiliensis natural-latex and Euphorbiaceae members. A brief summary of the study is as follows: Allergen cross-reactions among three strongly sensitizing Euphorbiaceae species, i.e., the rubber tree (Hevea brasiliensis), castor bean (Ricinus communis), and the Mediterranean weed Mercurialis annua were studied in Finnish patients (n = 25) allergic to Hevea brasiliensis natural-latex, but with no known exposure to castor bean or M. annua, and French patients allergic to castor bean (n = 26) or to M. annua (n = 9), but not to Hevea brasiliensis natural-latex. In immunoglobulin-E immunoblotting, 28 percent of Hevea brasiliensis natural-latex allergic patient sera recognized castor bean seed and 48 percent reacted to castor bean pollen proteins. Likewise, 35 percent of the Hevea brasiliensis natural-latex allergic patient sera bound to M. annua pollen allergens. Nineteen percent of castor bean-allergic patients showed immunoglobulin-E to Hevea brasiliensis natural-latex and 8 percent to M. annua proteins. Sera from patients allergic to M. annua reacted in 44 percent to Hevea brasiliensis natural-latex, in 56 percent to castor bean seed, and in 78 percent to castor bean pollen proteins. In immunoblotting, castor bean seed extract inhibited the binding of Hevea brasiliensis natural-latex reactive immunoglobulin-E to 20 kDa, 30 kDa of Hevea brasiliensis natural-latex, and 55 kDa of proteins; Hevea brasiliensis natural-latex extract, in turn, inhibited the binding of castor bean-reactive immunoglobulin-E to 14, 21-22, 29, and 32-34 kDa of castor bean proteins. In enzyme-linked immunosorbent assay (ELISA) inhibition, Hevea brasiliensis natural-latex extract inhibited 33 percent of the binding of M. annua--reactive immunoglobulin-E of pooled sera to M. annua pollen. In conclusion, allergen cross-reactivity in vitro was observed among three botanically related Euphorbiaceae members, H. brasiliensis, R. communis, and M. annua, but the molecular specificity of the observed cross-reactions as well as their clinical significance remains to be elucidated. Allergen cross-reactivity should be taken into account in diagnostic work [11].

Mold

Research has shown that there is a cross reaction between Hevea brasiliensis natural-latex and mold. A brief summary of the study is as follows: Hevea brasiliensis natural-latex allergy is an immunoglobulin-E mediated disease that is caused by proteins that elute from commercial latex products. A complementary DNA (cDNA) coding for *Hev-b* 9, an enolase (2-phospho-D-glycerate hydrolyase) and allergen from latex of the rubber tree Hevea brasiliensis was amplified by PCR. The PCR primers were designed according to conserved regions of enolases from plants. The obtained cDNA amplification product consisted of 1651 bp and encoded a protein of 445 amino-acid residues with a calculated molecular mass of 47.6 kDa. Sequence comparisons revealed high similarities of the Hevea latex enolase to mold enolases that have been identified as important allergens. In addition, the crucial amino-acid residues that participate in the formation of the catalytic site and the $Mg2+$ binding site of enolases were also conserved. Hevea latex enolase was produced as a recombinant protein in Escherichia coli with an N-terminal hexahistidyl tag, and purified by affinity chromatography. The yield amounted to 110 mg of purified *Hev-b* 9 per litre of bacterial culture. The recombinant allergen bound immunoglobulin-E from latex, as well as mold-allergic patients, in immunoblot and ELISA experiments. The natural enolase was isolated from Hevea latex by (NH4)2SO4 precipitation and ion exchange chromatography. The natural and the recombinant (r)*Hev-b* 9 showed equivalent enzymatic activity. Patients' immunoglobulin-E antibodies preincubated with r*Hev b-* 9 lost their ability to bind to natural (n) *Hev-b* 9, indicating the identity of the B-cell epitopes on both molecules. Cross-reactivity with two enolases from Cladosporium herbarum and Alternaria alternata was determined by inhibition of immunoglobulin-E binding to these enolases by *rHev-b* 9. Therefore, enolases may represent another class of highly conserved enzymes with allergenic potentials [12].

Mold induced asthma can cause a child to have an asthma attack that could be severe enough to require immediate medical attention.

Vegetables

Research has shown that there is a cross reaction between Hevea brasiliensis natural-latex and vegetables. A brief summary of the study is as follows: A study that evaluated 1,3-B-glucanases as candidates in latex-pollen-vegetable food cross-reactivity. The aim of this work was to study the potential implication of 1,3-β-glucanases in cross-reactivity among latex, pollen and vegetable foods. The research showed that cDNA encoding the N-terminal domain and homologous glucanases are new molecules to be used in diagnostic protocols as they could help to identify allergic pollen patients who are at risk for developing allergic symptoms to fruits, vegetables and latex [13].

Insect Venoms

Research has shown that there is a cross reaction between Hevea brasiliensis natural-latex and insect venom. A brief summary of the study is as follows: The study investigated whether there are cross-reactive immunoglobulin-E binding structures in Hevea brasiliensis natural-latex and hymenoptera venoms. The research showed that insect venoms and Hevea brasiliensis natural-latex share immunoglobulin-E binding CCD that may be responsible for positive serological test results to Hevea brasiliensis natural-latex in patients with insect venom allergy. This occurs frequently (13.6 percent) among venom-allergic individuals and did not elicit clinical symptoms upon contact to Hevea brasiliensis natural-latex in the patients examined. In contrast, true co-sensitization to insect venoms and Hevea brasiliensis natural-latex allergens can occur and may not be missed [14].

Grass & Weed Pollen

Research has shown that Hevea brasiliensis natural-latex, grass pollen, and weed pollen share immunoglobulin-E epitopes [15].

Sugar Beets

A study has shown that a sugar beet gene is related to the latex allergen *Hev-b* 5 family. The research showed that the protein encoded by this gene was found to be alanine-rich and glutamic acid-rich and that it resembles members of the latex allergen *Hev-b* 5 family [16].

Fruits

The following information is from the Vanderbilt University Medical-Center website describing Hevea brasiliensis natural-latex and food allergies. Existing or potential food allergies should be considered in any person with an allergic reaction to Hevea brasiliensis natural-latex. Persons allergic/sensitive to Hevea brasiliensis natural-latex may react to all, some, or none of the cross-reactive foods. The food sensitivity may exist before, at the same time or after the development of Hevea brasiliensis natural-latex sensitivity. It is, therefore, recommended that the foods described below be avoided to prevent the development of cross-reactions. Example of cross react foods to Hevea brasiliensis natural-latex and the degree of association are as follows:

High Association: Banana; Avocado; Kiwi; and Chestnut.

As an example, a study has shown that large numbers of children are developing severe allergies to kiwifruit. Researchers from the University of South Hampton studied 273 adults and children suspected of having an allergy to the popular fruit, with 45 subjects undergoing testing. Until now little has been known about the numbers of people allergic to the fruit. One in five subjects suffered severe symptoms including collapse, wheezing and vomiting. Researchers found that 40% of cases occurred in children, a pattern not found with other frequently allergenic foods, such as dairy foods or peanuts. The research also stated, "Curiously, kiwifruit proteins have the same composition as the raw Malaysian rubber used to make latex gloves, balloons and condoms, and those allergic to either kiwifruit or latex experience similar reactions." Almost all (90 percent) of the children under six in the study had an underlying condition such as hay fever, eczema or asthma, and 60% reported having a peanut allergy [17].

Moderate Association: Apple; Carrot; Celery; Tomato; Papaya; Potato; and Melon.

As an example, a study has shown that allergy to cooked potatoes is a cause of severe allergic disease, with immediate reactions and eczema in some atopic infants and young children [18]. It has been speculated that the consumption of French fries may be involved in the atypicality of Autism Spectrum Disorders. As an example, there was a lawsuit filed in Los Angeles California that claimed McDonald's french fries caused an autistic child to suffer from tantrums and digestive problems. According to a lawsuit, after eating French fries at a McDonald's in Valencia, Calif., the child experienced increased aggression and tantrums, while his ability to communicate and take care of himself diminished. Potato allergy may have been an issue but the culprits, according to the suit, were gluten and casein - ingredients found in milk and wheat products - and which some parents of autistic children believe can exacerbate the condition. McDonald's has acknowledged that its hash browns and french fries, historically reported as allergen-free, may in fact contain wheat and milk ingredients from the oil they are cooked in.

Low Association: Pear; Peach; Cherry; Pineapple; Strawberry; Grape; Hazelnut; Walnut; fig; Peanut; Rye; Wheat; Apricot; and Nectarine [19].

Tobacco

Prohevein-like defense protein of tobacco is a cross-reactive allergen for latex-allergic patients [20].

Peanuts

Analysis of the *Hev-b* proteins has revealed a similarity to the Early Nodule Specific Protein of leguminous plants [21]. A life-threatening reaction to peanut allergies can be anaphylaxis. This causes constriction of airways that can stop breathing completely or makes it very difficult. Also, the throat can swell, shock can occur, blood pressure can drop dangerously, the pulse becomes rapid, and often the person becomes dizzy, lightheaded or unconscious. This is a medical emergency requiring immediate treatment.

It is important to know that natural-latex allergy can go into remission from reduced exposure, while induced cross-react allergies to homologous proteins in fruits and vegetables may remain persistent based on repeated exposure to such foods. Thus, the after effects of natural-latex allergy may continue to stress adaptive immunity long after the natural-latex allergy has gone into remission.

There is growing evidence that dissimilar proteins can complex and be recognized as an antigen. For example, research has shown that hormones may combine with dissimilar proteins resulting in a protein-protein complex that may be recognized as foreign. Thereafter, the hormone part of the molecule complex may be recognized as an antigen [22].

The deliberate commingling of food stuff proteins and natural-latex may affect the incidence of cross-reactions. As an example, corn starch is a non-homologous polymer that has been associated with natural- latex. Corn-starch powder has been used as a slip aid in the manufacture of natural-latex based gloves. It is known that the proteins in natural-latex can migrate from the glove and onto the corn-starch. The protein contaminated powder readily becomes air-borne and increases exposure through inhalation [23]. In a theoretical model of a cross-react immune response, the commingling of corn-starch and natural-latex may induce dendritic cells to present amylase and antigenic protein fragments. Thereafter, memory-b cells may then recognition carbohydrates based on amylase and glucose homology. Specifically, amylose in corn-starch has similar ring-size glucose units and glycosidic linkage configuration to maltose.

Another example where food stuff proteins are deliberately commingled with natural-latex is in water-based adhesives. Specifically, the milk protein casein is often added to natural- latex adhesives as a thickening agent (i.e. rheology modifier). Consumer groups have sought warning labels on food packaging containing natural-latex adhesives, saying the substance poses a potential threat to people with allergic sensitivities [24]. The deliberate commingling of food-stuff proteins with natural-latex should be prohibited in an effort to reduce the global incidence and prevalence of food allergies. Research efforts should be initiated using protein-protein docking techniques to predict protein commingling interactions to determine if such an interaction affects the cross-react mechanism.

Natural-latex exposure is increasing the prevalence of allergies, is it reasonable to ask these questions?

[5] Are the allergenic proteins or the unclassified allergenic proteins within natural-latex becoming more allergenic based on structure change through molecular evolution?

[6] Are future generations becoming more sensitive to the allergenic proteins or the unclassified proteins within natural-latex based on inherited immunity?

[7] Does the prevalence of diseases within natural-latex affect the allergenic protein characteristics? Examples of diseases include Rigidoporus, Pink Disease, South American leaf blight, Corynespora leaf fall disease, Colletotrichum leaf fall, Red root disease, Collar rot, Brown rot, Black crust disease, and Black strip.

In Germany, studies on the hazards of certain natural-latex based medical products have initiated Government regulations restricting their usage. For example, regulation TRGS 540 enacted in 1998 banned the use of all powdered gloves in German health care facilities. In the United States, Johns Hopkins Hospital has banned nearly all natural-latex products. The landmark Baltimore hospital where natural-latex gloves were invented has become the first major medical institution to ban such natural-latex products [25].

Efforts have been made to commercialize alternative latex having inherently lower antigenic protein content (i.e., guayule rubber latex and the Russian dandelion) but such materials are reported to be higher in cost and presently are available only in limited quantities. Furthermore, both of these materials have their own unique set of proteins with potential allergenic behavior not yet clearly understood. For example, a guayule rubber producing plant having inherently reduced protein content is currently being evaluated as a potential hypoallergenic alternative. The major protein in guayule rubber (approximately fifty percent protein total) is cytochrome P-450 which has been shown to have about twenty five percent homology to human cytochrome P-450. There are more than 12,000 plant species that yield latex containing rubber, though in the vast majority of those species the rubber is not suitable for commercial use [26].

Other efforts are being made to deproteinize Hevea brasiliensis natural-latex to help reduce natural-latex allergies. As an example, a biotechnology corporation located in Duluth, Georgia is leading the way by inventing protein removal methods that significantly reduce the amount of proteins in Hevea brasiliensis natural-latex adhesives.

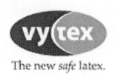

The new *safe* latex.

Vystar Corporation has developed Vytex®-Natural rubber latex (NRL) which is a new product designed to offer a standardized source material for the production of natural rubber products using chemically modified Hevea brasiliensis natural-latex to significantly reduce its antigenic protein content. The method of protein removal is achieved by the introduction of aluminum hydroxide which has well known protein binding characteristics. The insoluble aluminum hydroxide-protein complex is separated from the aqueous natural- latex dispersion by filtration or centrifugation to provide an Ultra Low-Protein Hevea brasiliensis natural-latex product. The multi-patented Vytex™-NRL process effectively removes proteins to virtually undetectable levels as determined by independent testing using two industry standard methodologies; Modified Lowry (American Society for Testing and Materials D5712) for total proteins and ELISA (American Society for Testing and Materials D6499) measuring antigenic protein levels. Over 500 medical and non-medical products made with Vytex™-NRL have been independently tested using accredited American Society for Testing and Materials protein test methodologies. Vystar Corporation states that Vytex™-NRL consistently contains less than 10 μg/dm² of antigenic protein in unleached cast films – this level is considered safe by organizations setting industry standards including the *Malaysian Rubber Export Promotion Council* – SMG Certification Program (less than 50 μg/dm² of antigenic protein for powder-free gloves; Association of peri-Operative Registered Nurses (AORN), the 2004 AORN Latex Guidelines defines a latex safe environment if product protein content is less than 50 μg/dm² of total protein pursuant to American Society for

Testing and Materials D5712 and less than 10 µg/dm² of antigenic protein using the American Society for Testing and Materials D6499 antigen test. Furthermore, Vystar Corporation states that products made with Vytex®-NRL have dramatically reduced antigenic protein values up to ninety-nine percent, over standard Hevea brasiliensis natural-latex, and can be used for making surgical and examination gloves, condoms, foam, tubing, breather bags, balloons, adhesives as well as many other natural-latex based products across a wide range of industries. Recently, Vystar Corporation and Alatech Healthcare, LLC announced 510(k) clearance from the United States Food and Drug Administration to market and sell Alatech's Envy™ condom manufactured with Vytex™-NRL. The Envy™ condom will be the first medical product available in the United States made from Vystar's patented Vytex™-NRL which has less than 2 micrograms/dm² of the antigenic protein. Ultra low-protein natural-latex could be one of the most important health and safety initiatives of the 21ˢᵗ century.

REFERENCES

[1] The International Rubber Research and Development Board. Latex Protein Allergy:The Political Dimension. http://www.irrdb.com/irrdb/naturalrubber/latexallergy/causesoflatex.htm

[2] Swanson MC, Olsen D. (2000), Latex allergen affinity for starch powders applied to natural rubber latex gloves and released as an aerosol: From dust to don. *Journal of Allergy & Clinical Immunology, Vol. 5*, No 8.

[3] NIOSH Publication No. 97-135 (1997). Preventing Allergic Reactions to Natural Rubber Latex in the Workplace. http://www.cdc.gov/niosh/latexalt.html

[4] Yassin MS, Lierl MB, Fisher TJ, *et al.* (1994). Latex allergy in hospitals employees. *Ann Allergy. Vol. 72*, pp. 245-249.

[5] Benjamin B. Hayes, Aliakbar Afshari, Lyndell Millecchia, Patsy A. *et al.* (2000). Evaluation of Percutaneous Penetration of Natural Rubber Latex Proteins. *Toxicological Sciences. Vol. 56*, pages 262-270.

[6] Stephen Barlas. (1999). Rubber hits the Road at FDA. *Packaging World Magazine*. May, page 87.

[7] MC Dieguez Pastor, M Anton Girones, R Blanco, *et al.* (2006). Latex allergy in children - a follow-up study. *Allergologia et immunopathologia, Domingo L Enero. Volume 34*, Number 01, pages 17-22.

[8]   Wright HT, Brooks DM, Wright CS. (1985). Evolution of the multidomain protein wheat germ agglutinin. *Journal of Molecular Evolution. Vol.21*, pages 133-138.

[9]   T.Skovsted, B. Hansen, P. Staun-Olsen, et al. (2000). Demonstration of IgE cross reaction between latex and pine wood - a case report. ICACI, Sydney Austrailia, Oct. 15-20.

[10]   Ann-Therese Karlberg, Kerstin Magnusson. (1996). Rosin components identified in diapers, *Contact Dermatitis. Vol. 34*, pages 176-180.

[11]   Palosuo T, Panzani RC, Singh AB, *et al.* (2000). Allergen cross-reactivity between proteins of the latex from Hevea brasiliensis, seeds and pollen of Ricinus communis, and pollen of Mercurialis annua, members of the Euphorbiaceae family. *Allergy Asthma Proc. Vol. 23*, No. 2, pages 141-147.

[12]   Wagner S, Breiteneder H, Simon-Nobbe B, *et al.* (2000). Hev b 9, an enolase and a new cross-reactive allergen from hevea latex and molds. Purification, characterization, cloning and expression. *Eur. J. Biochem. Vol. 267*, pages 7006–7014.

[13]   Palomares O, Villalba M, Quiralte J, Polo F, *et al.* (2005). 1,3-B-glucanases as candidates in latex-pollen-vegetable food cross-reactivity. *Clinical & Experimental Allergy. Vol. 35*, page 345.

[14]   V. Mahler, C. Gutgesell, R. Valenta, *et al.* (2006). Natural Rubber Latex and hymenoptera venoms share Immunoglobin-E epitopes accounting for cross-reactive carbohydrate determinants. *Clin. Exp. Allergy. Vol. 35*, No. 11, pages 1446-1456.

[15]   Fuchst T., Spitzauer S., Vente C., *et al.* (1997). Natural Latex, grass pollen, weed pollen share IgE epitopes. *Journal of Allergy and Clinical Immunology. Vol. 100*, No. 3, pages 356-64.

[16]   Mark R. Fowler, Jill Gartland, William Norton, et al. (2000). RS2 - a sugar beet gene related to the latex allergen *Hev-b* 5 family. *Journal of Experimental Botany. Vol. 51*, No. 353, pages 2125-2126.

[17]   The Sunday Herald. News Publication. Children develop allergy to favorite fruit. June 27, 2004, http://findarticles.com/p/articles/mi_qn 4156/is_20040627/ai_n12589546/

[18]   De Swert LF, Cadot P, Ceuppens JL. (2002). Allergy to cooked white potatoes in infants and young children: A cause of severe, chronic allergic disease. *Journal of Allergy Clinical Immunology. Vol. 110*, No. 3, pages 524-535.

[19] Vanderbilt University Medical Center: Latex and Food Allergies; the
      Protein   Connection.   http://www.mc.vanderbilt.edu/pcs/quality/latex/
      nutrition.html
[20] Hanninen AR, Kalkkinen N, Mikkola JH, Helin J, *et al.* (2000). Prohevein-
      like defense protein of tobacco is a cross-reactive allergen for latex-allergic
      patients. *Journal of Allergy Clinical Immunology. Vol. 106*, No. 4, pages
      778-779.
[21] Yeang Hoong Yeet. (2003). Malaysia Rubber Board, and Science: Hunting
      for   the   elusive   latex   allergen.   http://www.lgm.gov.my/rubnews
      /2003/rub250303.html
[22] Medical News Today. (2006). Evidence of estrogen and progesterone
      hormone allergy has been discovered by research in Texas.
      http://www.medicalnewstoday.com/articles/40717.php
[23] Public Citizen. (1998). American Society of Health-System Pharmacists,
      Ban Proposed for Latex Gloves Powdered with Cornstarch. http://www.
      tradewatch.org/pressroom/release.cfm?ID=142
[24] Consumeraffairs.com. (2006). Latex in Food Packaging Poses Risk
      www.consumeraffairs.com/news04/2006/08/latex.html.
[25] physorg.com. (2008). Latex banned at Johns Hopkins Hospital.
      http://www.physorg.com/news119886779.html.
[26] Bowers, J.E. (1990). Natural Rubber-Producing Plants for the United States.
      Beltsville, MD: National Agricultural Library. Pages 1-3.

Chapter IV

ADAPTIVE IMMUNITY

It is not the strongest of the species that survives, nor the most intelligent, but the ones most responsive to change. – Charles Darwin

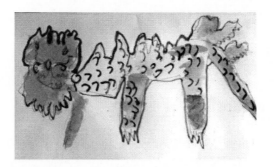

Dain's pediatrician removed the natural-latex protective gloves from his hands after completing the examination. A wisp of powder floated into the air as the gloves were peeled off his hands and discarded into a waste basket next to the examination table. The pediatrician's eyes extensively scanned and sorted through several years of routine examinations. The silence that filled the room was interrupted by Dain's self calming hum as he strenuously rocked back and forth on the examination table. It was clear that Dain had dramatically regressed over the last several months. A forty word vocabulary was completely gone and social interactions were now replaced with repetitive self-stimulation. Dain's well defined muscles, on both arms and legs, gave an indication of the repetitive jumping and flapping behaviors which seemed to increase daily. Three to four hours of sleep per night seemed to provide more than enough rest, his mind and body were now in constant hyper-drive. With a sudden certainty in his expression and voice the pediatrician looked up from the clipboard and said, "Dain's symptoms indicate that he may have Autism and I can't help you any further". The parents' attention and eyes were on Dain. The pediatrician dug into his pocket pulling out a prescription notepad. He quickly scribbled a name and number on the pad and handed it to the parents and said, "This person can get Dain an official diagnosis". Although Dain could hear everything around him, his mind understood nothing that was being said.

WHY HAVE NATURAL-LATEX ALLERGENS BEEN DRAMATICALLY PRESENTED OVER THE LAST THIRTY YEARS?

Medical science now recognizes that the use of powdered natural-latex gloves, wherein the allergens absorb onto the powder and become airborne, has significantly contributed to the incidence of allergies (Iatrogenic allergies).

Allergies fall within 4 specific groups:

Type I Hypersensitivity

Type I hypersensitivity or immediate hypersensitivity, immunoglobulin-E antibodies cause an allergic reaction provoked by re-exposure to a specific type of antigen referred to as an allergen. Exposure may be by ingestion, inhalation, injection, or direct contact. This includes things like hay fever, food allergies, pet danger allergies, and medication allergies, among others. Any allergy that causes a fast reaction, whether it's sneezing, scratching or even a severe reaction like anaphylactic shock falls into this group. Type I allergies are the most common of all the allergies.

Type II Hypersensitivity

In type II hypersensitivity, the immunoglobulin-M and immunoglobulin-G antibodies produced by the immune response bind to antigens on the patient's own cell surfaces. The antigens recognized in this way may either be intrinsic ("self" antigen, innately part of the patient's cells) or extrinsic (absorbed onto the cells during exposure to some foreign antigen. These cells are recognized by macrophages or dendritic cells which act as antigen presenting cells; this causes a B-cell response where antibodies are produced against the foreign antigen.

Type III Hypersensitivity

In type III hypersensitivity immune complex occurs when antigens and antibodies such as immunoglobulin-G or immunoglobulin-M are present in roughly equal amounts, causing extensive cross-linking. It is characterized by soluble antigens that are not bound to cell surfaces. When the antigens and antibodies bind together large immune complexes are formed. They deposit in tissues and induce an inflammatory response and can cause damage wherever they precipitate. The reaction can take hours, days, or even weeks to develop.

Type IV Hypersensitivity

Type IV hypersensitivity is often called delayed type hypersensitivity in that the reaction takes two to three days to develop. This type of allergy is also called a cellular immune reaction (T-cells).

Are Autism Spectrum Disorders the pro-creativity of Immunity?

Allergy induced Autism is an area of research wherein immune responses to certain environmental proteins, and foodstuff proteins, may affect the development and intensity of atypical behaviors within the Autism Spectrum.

The allergens in natural-latex are known to cause severe and pervasive immune responses. In children, repeated exposure to such allergens has been shown to cause an increased incidence of sensitization, adverse allergic reactions, and even death through anaphylactic shock. Natural-latex has seen a dramatic increase in usage over the last 30-years (e.g., health care industry, consumer products). The timing, frequency, intensity, and type of exposure to such proteins may influence the incidence, degree of atypicality, and prevalence of Autism Spectrum Disorders. Research efforts are exploring how immune responses to such proteins affect lymphocyte sensitivity, enzyme regulation, and neural formation during prenatal/neonatal/infant development [1].

It is now well understood that all of us have the potential for allergies based on the presence of immunoglobulin-E antibodies which are part of the adaptive immune system. The frequency of exposure to allergenic proteins may influence the prevalence of an allergy. For example, a primary challenge to antigenic proteins may induce the activation of virgin T & B cells, and long lived memory T & B cells. Thereafter, repeated exposures to such proteins re-activate existing memory T & B cells and stimulate further production of T & B cells (i.e., virgin cells and memory cells).

How can Allergies Affect brain Development?

Neuron growth factor is a protein critical for the survival and maintenance of sympathetic and sensor neurons, and lymphocyte expression. The 1986 Nobel Prize in Medicine was awarded to Stanley Cohen and Rita Levi-Montalcini for work showing that neuron growth factor is an extremely potent biological substance for the growth of sensory and sympathetic nerves. The discovery of nerve growth factor in the beginning of the 1950's is a fascinating example of how a skilled observer can create a concept out of apparent chaos. Until this time, experimental neurobiologists did not understand how the development of the nervous system was regulated to result in the final complete innervations of the body. The investigation of neuron growth factor's role in the development of the nervous system, as well as later, in adult neural function, has been a lifelong dedication for Rita Levi-Montalcini. Developmental biologist Rita Levi-Montalcini, who in the beginning of 1950's moved from her homeland Italy, to Viktor Hamburger's laboratory in St. Louis, USA, showed in 1952 that when tumors from mice were transplanted to chick embryos they induced potent growth of the chick embryo nervous system, specifically sensory and sympathetic nerves. Since this outgrowth did not require direct contact between the tumor and the chick embryo, Rita Levi-Montalcini concluded that the tumor released a nerve growth-promoting factor which had a selective action on certain types of nerves. Following this discovery, Rita Levi-Montalcini turned to a more sensitive cell culture system in order to measure neuron growth factor activity in various extracts. Neuron growth factor proved to be an extremely potent biological substance. A sensory or sympathetic nerve cell reacted within 30 seconds to the addition of minute quantities of neuron growth factor. One billionth part of a gram of neuron growth factor per ml of culture medium exerted a potent growth-promoting effect. A few minutes after the addition of neuron growth factor, nerve fibres began to grow out from the ganglion which after a day's exposure to neuron growth factor resembled a sun surrounded by rays. This biological assay to detect neuron growth factor paved the way for the next step in this pathway of discovery - identification of the active nerve growth-promoting substance. The recent finding of neuron growth factor in the brain has raised great expectation. An important pathway in the brain with acetylcholine as a transmitter substance seems to be sensitive to neuron growth factor [2].

A study has shown that circulating neuron growth factor levels are increased in humans with allergic diseases. Nerve growth factor serum levels were measured in 49 patients with asthma and/or rhino-conjunctivitis and/or urticaria-angioedema. Clinical and biochemical parameters, such as bronchial reactivity, total and specific serum immunoglobulin-E levels, and circulating eosinophil cationic protein levels, were evaluated in relation to neuron growth factor values in asthma patients. Neuron growth factor was significantly increased in the 42 allergic (skin-test- or radio-allergosorbent-test-positive) subjects (49.7 +/- 28.8 pg/ml) versus the 18 matched controls (3.8 +/- 1.7 pg/ml; P < 0.001). Neuron growth factor levels in allergic patients with asthma, rhino-conjunctivitis, and urticaria-angioedema were 132.1 +/- 90.8, 17.6 +/- 6.1, and 7.6 +/- 1.8 pg/ml (P < 0.001, P < 0.002, and P < 0.05 versus controls), respectively. Patients with more than one allergic disease had higher neuron growth factor serum values than those with a single disease. When asthma patients were considered as a group, neuron growth factor serum values (87.6 +/- 59.8 pg/ml) were still significantly higher than those of control groups (P < 0.001), but allergic asthma patients had elevated neuron growth factor serum levels compared with nonallergic asthma patients (132.1 +/- 90.8 versus 4.9 +/- 2.9 pg/ml; P < 0.001). Neuron growth factor serum levels correlate to total immunoglobulin-E serum values (rho = 0.43; P < 0.02). The highest neuron growth factor values were found in patients with severe allergic asthma, a high degree of bronchial hyper-reactivity, and high total immunoglobulin-E and eosinophil cationic protein serum levels. This study represents the first observation (that we know of) that neuron growth factor is increased in human allergic inflammatory diseases and asthma [3].

Furthermore, increased levels of neuron growth factor have been shown to induce growth and differentiation of human B lymphocytes (B-cells). The principal functions of B-cells are to make antibodies against antigens, perform the role of Antigen Presenting Cells and eventually develop into memory B-cells after activation by antigen interaction. B-cells are an essential component of the adaptive immune system [4].

Neuron growth factor expression has been linked to Autism. In a study, investigators examined and compared archived neonatal blood samples from children born in four northern California counties from 1983 to 1985 who later developed Autism, mental retardation, cerebral palsy or developed normally. The investigators measured concentrations of several neural growth factors and found that the growth factors were significantly elevated in the neonatal blood of children who later developed Autism or mental retardation, but not in the blood from children who developed cerebral palsy or blood from the normal controls [5].

Adding clarity to allergy induced Autism, the elimination of synapses (i.e., pruning) may be universal to all neural systems and that the patterned connections within the brain are based solely on large-scale regressive events. Pruning, in the absence of cell death, is thought to be influenced by the expression of neurotrophic factors including neuron growth factor [6].

Infant brains may be more susceptible to the expression of neuron growth factor in that the blood brain barrier is not fully developed compared to adults. It is speculated that in allergy induced Autism, the over-expression of neuron growth factor during prenatal/neonatal/infant development may affect the pruning mechanism resulting in over-connectivity.

Recent studies indicate over-connectivity in Autism Spectrum Disorders. Specifically, a review highlighted neurobiological findings during the first years of life and emphasizes early brain overgrowth as a key factor in the pathobiology of Autism. The research showed that excess neuron numbers may be one possible cause of early brain overgrowth and produce defects in neural patterning and wiring, with exuberant local and short-distance cortical interactions impeding the function of large-scale, long-distance interactions between brain regions. Because large-scale networks underlie socio-emotional and communication functions, such alterations in brain architecture could relate to the early clinical manifestations of Autism. As such, Autism may additionally provide unique insight into genetic and developmental processes that shape early neural wiring patterns and make possible higher-order social, emotional, and communication functions [7].

In a theoretical model, neonatal saliva testing may be a useful non-invasive medical procedure to determine if a child is experiencing the manifestations of allergy induced Autism. Neuron growth factor has been observed in human saliva. Thus, in the future this simple test could be used as a screening method to determine the likelihood of developing an Autism Spectrum Disorder [8].

Further research has shown that allergy may play a role in the pathogenesis of Autism wherein allergic immune responses to some proteins (e.g., natural-latex and dietary proteins) may induce the production of brain auto-antibodies, which are found in many autistic children. The study was conducted to investigate the frequency of allergic manifestations in autistic children. More specifically, the relationship between allergy and disease characteristics in terms of disease severity, clinical findings and electroencephalography abnormalities was also studied. Fifty autistic children (thirty had mild to moderate Autism and twenty had severe Autism) were studied in comparison to fifty age-and-sex matched children without neuro-psychiatric manifestations serving as controls. Clinical evaluation was done with special emphasis on neuro-psychiatric assessment and clinical manifestations of allergy. Serum total immunoglobulin E was measured in all studied subjects. In addition, electroencephalograph and assessment of mental age were done for all autistic children. Allergic manifestations (bronchial asthma, atopic dermatitis and/or allergic rhinitis) were found in fifty two percent of autistic patients. This frequency was significantly higher than that of controls (ten percent; $P < 0.001$). There was a significant positive association between the frequency of allergic manifestations and disease severity, important clinical findings elicited in some autistic children (gastrointestinal symptoms and neurological manifestations) and electroencephalograph abnormalities. The research showed that the frequency of allergic manifestations is increased in autistic children. The significant positive association between these manifestations and important disease characteristics (disease severity, gastrointestinal symptoms, neurological findings and electroencephalograph abnormalities) may shed light on the possible causal role of allergy in some autistic children. Indeed, we need to know more about the links between allergy, immune system and brain in Autism. This is important to determine whether therapeutic modulation of immune function and allergic diseases are legitimate avenues for novel therapy in selected cases of Autism or even for attempted primary prevention in genetically at risk subgroups [9].

Although there are many materials that may affect allergies in children, it is reasonable to assume that most allergenic materials have not substantially increased over the last thirty years. The immune responsive material that has dramatically presented itself over the last thirty years is the allergenic proteins inherent in natural-latex [10].

It has often been said that natural-latex allergy usually affects people who are routinely exposed to natural-latex. Many neonates are routinely exposed to baby bottle nipples and pacifiers that are formed from natural-latex. We are currently at the mercy of rubber manufacturers, many of which are located in third world countries; in that allergenic protein content is not mandated. Other natural-latex based articles that children are exposed to include diaper adhesives, mattresses, bed pads, balloons, teething articles, toys, rubber bands, pencil erasers, carpet padding and carpet adhesives, and food packaging adhesives. Johns Hopkins Researchers have encouraged the Food and Drug Administration and pharmaceutical companies to discontinue the use of natural-latex stoppers in medicinal vials. A single exposure may cause immune sensitivity.

Asia continues to dominate the world supply of natural-latex, averaging more than 90 percent of total world production. The largest natural-latex producing countries include Thailand, Indonesia and Malaysia. Thailand is currently the largest producer, but Indonesia is closing in on Thai natural-latex production, and is expected to overtake Thai production in coming years. Malaysia, which accounted for 32 percent of world production in 1988, shifted emphasis to other crops and non-agricultural investments and produced only 8 percent of the world total by 1998. Today, Malaysia represents roughly 12 percent of total world natural-latex production. Other regions that are expecting high growth in natural-latex production include Brazil, Guatemala, India, Sri Lanka, the Philippines and Vietnam.

The world's three largest importers of natural-latex are China, the United States of America, and Japan. In continuation, these countries have reported that the incidence of Autism Spectrum Disorders is also increasing at an alarming rate.

In the United States, the largest user of natural-latex is the state of Ohio. Researcher's have reported over a six thousand percent increase in Autism Spectrum Disorders in Ohio from 1992-1999. Other states that have seen dramatic increases include Oregon, Minnesota, and Maine all of which have industries that are significant users of natural-latex [11].

Although products formed from natural-latex are used extensively around the world, the primary producers and users described above may be experiencing an increased incidence of allergy induced Autism due to increased exposure.

In the other extreme, communities that are less likely to use or be exposed to products formed from natural-latex have shown an astonishingly low Autism rate. For example, the Autism Spectrum Disorders rate for Amish around Middlefield, Ohio, is 1 in 15,000. Research has found scant evidence of Autism Spectrum

Disorders among sizable Amish settlements in Indiana and Kentucky [12]. Atopy in a United States Amish population has been studied. Sib-pair analysis of one-hundred seventy individuals from eleven Amish families revealed evidence for linkage of five markers in chromosome 5q31.1 with a gene controlling total serum immunoglobulin-E. The study suggests that immunoglobulin-E or a nearby gene in 5q31.1 regulates immunoglobulin-E production in a nonantigen-specific (non-cognate) fashion indicating that the Amish population is not resistant to allergies [13].

Factors that influence the incidence of allergy induced Autism include timing, frequency, intensity, and type of exposure:

Timing

The *Children's Environmental Health Centers,* which is funded by the United States Environmental Protection Agency, states in their website, "For many reasons, children are likely to be more vulnerable than adults to the effects of environmental contaminants. To better understand the effects of these exposures on children's health, the Centers for Children's Environmental Health and Disease Prevention Research ("Children's Centers") were established to explore ways to reduce children's health risks from environmental factors."

Research shows that the central nervous system is known to be susceptible to environmental insult (e.g., toxins and allergens) especially during prenatal/neonatal/infant development. The central nervous system is particularly vulnerable at this stage in that there is a proliferation of nerve cell reproduction, growth, and migration [14].

Furthermore, allergen exposure and sensitization during pregnancy has been shown to favor the development of atopy in the neonate. As an example, a study analyzed the impact of maternal immune responses on onset and subsequent development of allergen-specific immunity and immediate-type hypersensitivity in early childhood. The research showed that immunity present during pregnancy has a decisive impact on shaping of the Th1/Th2 T-cell profile in the neonate [15].

Repeated exposure to allergenic proteins during pregnancy may affect the genetic code of immune cells making the fetus more susceptible to allergies [16]. Maternal and infant exposure to natural-latex has often occurred in medical hospitals during visits/examinations. In a study on natural-latex hypersensitivity:

an iatrogenic and occupational risk; research showed that immediate hypersensitivity reactions from natural-latex products pose a significant threat to patients, healthcare workers, and the general population [17]. Hospitals have made efforts to eliminate such products but there remains much litigation and the evidence of harm is well documented, especially in the health care industry [18].

Is there a Historical Connection of Natural-Latex Exposure and allergy induced Autism?

The Hungarian physician Ignace Semmelweis discovered by 1847 that the incidence of puerperal fever could be drastically cut by the use of hand washing standards in obstetrical clinics. Many years thereafter, the germ theory of disease developed and displaced dyscrasia as the cause of many diseases. Ironically, medical hygiene products like natural-latex gloves that are intended to protect the practitioner and patient from infectious insult has increased non-infectious protein insult inducing allergies.

In a study on a retrospective analysis of risk factors in development of natural-latex allergy in children up to 5 years of age; the research showed that besides the number of operations and an atopic predisposition, no other definite risk factor for developing sensitization or allergy to natural-latex, such as everyday household objects, can be identified in children up to 5 years of age [19].

William Stewart Halsted who was Johns Hopkins Hospital's first surgeon in chief is widely credited as the first to develop and introduce natural-latex surgical gloves in 1894 which was five years after the institution opened.

The first mention of natural-latex allergy in a medical journal was in 1933. Dr. John G. Downing described two surgeons who came to him complaining of hand dermatitis after wearing rubber gloves during surgery [20].

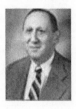

Leo Kanner

In 1930 Dr. Leo Kanner developed the first child psychiatry service in a pediatric center at Johns Hopkins hospital, Baltimore. Thereafter, the classification of Autism occurred in 1943 by the same person in the same hospital. Eleven children with striking behavioral similarities were given the label "Early Infantile Autism".

Thus, it appears that the timing of the discovery of natural-latex allergy and Autism coincide in medical history.

At about the same time, an Austrian scientist named Dr. Hans Asperger made similar observations. As described in Wikipedia:

> Asperger published the first definition of Asperger syndrome in 1944. In four boys, he identified a pattern of behavior and abilities that he called "autistic psychopathy", meaning Autism (self) and psychopathy (personality disease). The pattern included "a lack of empathy, little ability to form friendships, one-sided conversation, intense absorption in a special interest, and clumsy movements." Asperger called children with AS "little professors" because of their ability to talk about their favorite subject in great detail. It is commonly said that the paper was based on only four boys, however, Dr. Günter Krämer, of Zürich, who knew Asperger, states that it "was based on investigations of more than 400 children".
>
> Asperger was convinced that many of the children he identified as having autistic symptoms would use their special talents in adulthood. He followed one child, Fritz V., into adulthood. Fritz V. became a professor of astronomy and solved an error in Newton's work he originally noticed as a child. Hans Asperger's positive outlook contrasts strikingly with Leo Kanner's description of Autism, of which Asperger's is often considered to be a high-functioning form. In his 1944 paper, Asperger wrote:
>
> "We are convinced, then, that autistic people have their place in the organism of the social community. They fulfill their role well, perhaps better than anyone else could, and we are talking of people who as children had the greatest difficulties and caused untold worries to their care-givers."
>
> Near the end of World War II, Asperger opened a school for children with autistic psychopathy, with Sister Victorine. The school was bombed towards the end of the war, Sister Victorine was killed, the school was destroyed and much of Hans Asperger's early work was lost. It was this

event that arguably delayed the understanding of Autism Spectrum conditions in the west.

Interestingly, as a child, Hans Asperger appears to have exhibited features of the very condition named after him. He was described as a remote and lonely child, who had difficulty making friends. He was talented in language; in particular he was interested in the Austrian poet Franz Grillparzer, whose poetry he would frequently quote to his uninterested classmates. He also liked to quote himself and often referred to himself from a third-person perspective.

Asperger died before his identification of this pattern of behavior became widely recognized, because his work was mostly in German and barely translated. The term "Asperger's syndrome" was popularized in a 1981 paper by British researcher Lorna Wing, which challenged the previously accepted model of Autism presented by Leo Kanner in 1943 Unlike Kanner, Hans Asperger's findings were ignored and disregarded in the English-speaking world in his lifetime. Finally, from the early 1990s, his findings began to gain notice, and nowadays Asperger syndrome is recognized as a diagnosis in a large part of the world.

International Asperger's Day, February 18, marks the anniversary of Hans Asperger's birth. International Asperger's Day was conceived by Asperger Services Australia.

One of Asperger's patients was Austrian writer and Nobel Prize in Literature laureate Elfriede Jelinek [21].

Frequency

The frequency of exposure to the allergen in natural-latex continues to rise. The main driving force of the faster growth rate of the latter period was and still is the *Acquired Immune Deficiency Syndrome-Human Immunodeficiency Virus* threat and the consequent growing awareness of the need for protection, reflected in the rapid rise of demand for medical gloves, in particular, since the mid-1980s. Gloves were the main reason for the rising natural-latex uptake over the past 20 years.

The products formed from natural-latex and the industries they are used in are wide and varied, ranging from industrial, household, and medical. Twenty-five percent of the rubber used today comes from rubber trees while seventy-five percent are petroleum based (i.e., synthetic rubbers). Global conflicts, politics, and petroleum supplies continue to affect the price and availability of synthetic rubbers making the use of natural rubber more desirable. Over the past forty three years, the world natural-latex consumption has grown at an average of 4.2 percent per year, increasing to an estimated 925,000 tonnes in 2003. However, the growth was not smooth; natural-latex consumption had a slower growth period from 1960 to 1983, with an average growth rate of 2.1 percent per year and a faster growing period from 1984 to 2003, averaging 5.6 percent per year. In terms of actual tonnage the increase was 159,000 tonnes and 597,000 tonnes for the respective periods.

In industrialized societies, an example of a pervasive source of exposure to natural-latex is from automobile tires. A study has shown that tire dust from tread wear has been shown to be a route of exposure. The prevalence and severity of natural-latex allergy has increased dramatically in the last 15 years due to exposure to natural-latex products. Although historically this health risk has been elevated in hospital personnel and patients, a recent survey has indicated a significant potential risk for the general population. To obtain a wide-spread source for natural-latex exposure, tire debris was considered. The study searched for the presence of natural-latex allergens in passenger car and truck tire tread, in debris deposited from the atmosphere near a freeway, and in airborne particulate matter samples representative of the entire year 1993 at two sites in the Los Angeles basin (California). After extraction of the samples with phosphate buffered saline, a modified-ELISA inhibition assay was used to measure relative allergen potency and Western blot analysis were used to identify natural-latex allergens. The inhibition studies with the human immunoglobulin-E natural-latex assay revealed inhibition by the tire tread source samples and ambient freeway dust, as well as by control natural-latex sap and natural-latex glove extracts. Levels of extractable natural-latex allergen per unit of protein extracted were about two orders of magnitude lower for tire tread as compared to natural-latex gloves. Western blot analysis using binding of human immunoglobulin-E from natural-latex sensitive patients showed a band at 34-36 kDa in all tire and ambient samples. Long Beach and Los Angeles, California, air samples showed four additional bands between 50 and 135 kDa. Alternative Western blot analyses using rabbit immunoglobulin-G raised against natural-latex proteins showed a broad band at 30-50 kDa in all samples, with additional bands in the urban air samples similar to the immunoglobulin-E results. A natural-latex cross-reactive material was identified in mountain cedar. In conclusion, the natural-latex allergens present in sediment and airborne particulate material, derived from tire debris, and generated by heavy urban vehicle traffic could be important factors in producing natural-latex allergy and asthma symptoms associated with air pollution particles [22].

Furthermore, disposal of spent tires continues to be an environmental concern in that such materials are not easily recycled and disposal through incineration is often not cost effective due to the proper handling of pyrolytic byproducts including airborne particulate and toxic gases. Efforts have been made to find new uses for spent automobile tires wherein they are ground into crumb rubber and used as filler in gardens or as playground surfaces. Although such efforts are well intended, these practices continue to increase natural-latex exposure to the general population.

Intensity

Atopic children are likely to be more sensitive to the allergens in natural-latex. Exposing children to natural-latex can stimulate the adaptive immune system to form increased levels of immunoglobulin-E primed mast-cells and basophils that may bind to homologous endogenous and exogenous proteins that are essential for proper growth and development. The first time a child is exposed to the allergens large amounts of IgE antibodies are made if such proteins are recognized as foreign. These IgE antibodies then attach themselves to mast cells and basophils to form IgE primed cells. Thereafter, re-exposure to allergens cause the IgE primed cells bind to the allergens and release granules and powerful chemical mediators including histamine, proteases, chemotactic factors, cytokines, and metabolites of arachidonic acid (i.e., degranulation).

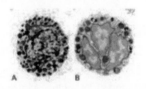

A = Human Mast Cell
B = Human Basophil

Type of Exposure

Natural-latex is used in many infant products including nipples for baby bottles, pacifiers, clothing, and toys. Routes of exposure may play an important role in determining sensitization.

A study has shown that differences in natural-latex specific immunoglobulin-E profiles and pulmonary function following sensitization of mice by four different routes suggest that exposure routes leading to sensitization may play a role in determining the primary allergens and the clinical manifestation of the immune response. The objective of the study was to evaluate the routes of sensitization in the development of natural-latex allergy using murine models representative of potential exposure routes by which health care workers (topical and respiratory) and spina bifida patients (subcutaneous) may be sensitized. BALB/c mice were administered Hevea brasiliensis natural-latex proteins by the subcutaneous, topical, intranasal, or intratracheal routes exhibited dose-responsive elevations in total immunoglobulin-E. *In vitro* splenocyte stimulation initially demonstrated specificity of the murine immune response to the Hevea brasiliensis natural-latex proteins. Subsequently, immuno-blot analysis was used to compare in Hevea brasiliensis natural-latex-specific immunoglobulin-E production amongst sensitization routes. Immuno-blots of immunoglobulin-E from subcutaneously sensitized mice demonstrated recognition of Hevea brasiliensis natural-latex proteins with molecular weights near 14 kDa and 27 kDa. These protein sizes are consistent with the molecular weights of major Hevea brasiliensis natural-latex allergens (*Hev b* 1 and *Hev b* 3). Mice sensitized by intratracheal or topical administration exhibited combined immunoglobulin-recognition of Hevea brasiliensis natural-latex proteins near 14 kDa, 35 kDa, and 92 kDa. These molecular weights are similar to other Hevea brasiliensis natural-latex allergens (*Hev b* 6, *Hev b* 2, and *Hev b* 4) commonly recognized by immunoglobulin-E of health care workers. Mice sensitized to Hevea brasiliensis natural-latex proteins by topical, intranasal, or intratracheal exposures exhibited bronco-constriction as evaluated by whole body plethysmography following respiratory challenge with such proteins [23].

The timing, frequency, intensity, and type of exposure to natural-latex can induce atypical immune responses and should be avoided during neurological development. The best means to eliminate the incidence of allergy induced Autism is natural-latex avoidance. All products coming into contact with children having a developing nervous system should be reviewed for natural-latex. Why?

Because the critical period for neurological development is from about three weeks to about sixteen weeks, although major structures of the brain continue to develop throughout childhood.

It has been speculated that natural-latex allergy may affect the incidence of Schizophrenia. A research paper has suggested that it cannot be denied that initial exposure to natural-latex in Europe occurred at exactly the same time that schizophrenia prevalence dramatically increased. It is also probable that sensitivity to natural-latex and schizophrenia are both associated with abnormal continuous oxidation of adrenalin to adrenochrome. The possibility exits, therefore, that schizophrenia is a consequence of natural-latex sensitivity [24].

In parallel, one of the five pervasive developmental disorders officially recognized by the American Psychiatric Association's Diagnostic and Statistical Manual of Mental Disorders is childhood disintegrative disorder, initially termed childhood schizophrenia.

The biochemist David Horrobin who was medical adviser to the Schizophrenia Association of Great Britain hypothesized that gene mutation is key to genius and despair and that Schizophrenia 'helped the ascent of man' [25].

In the future, medical science may determine which allergenic proteins affect neuro-cognitive development and these proteins will be excluded or introduced during critical stages of brain development. Thereafter, immunity and genius will continue to be part of man's journey -The intellectual movers and shakers of our society are atopic.

REFERENCES

[1]   M.J. Dochniak. "Autism Spectrum Disorders – Exogenous Protein Insult." *Med Hypotheses* (2007) Volume 69, Issue 3, page 545-549.

[2]   Nobelforsamlingen Kardinska Institutet Press Release -The Nobel Prize in Physiology or Medicine. (1986). Nobelforsamlingen Kardinska Institutet. http://nobelprize.org/nobel_prizes/medicine/laureates/1986/press.html

[3]   Sergio Bonini, Alessandro Lambiase, Stefano Bonini, *et al.* (1996). Circulating nerve growth factor levels are increased in humans with allergic diseases and asthma. *PNAS. Vol. 93*, Issue 20, pages 10955-10960.

[4]   Otten, U., Ehrhard, P., Peck, R. (1989). Nerve growth factor induces growth and differentiation of human B lymphocytes *Proc. Natl. Acad. Sci. Vol. 86*, pages 10059-10063.

[5] UniSci Article. (2001). Neuron Growth Factor Proteins Present At Birth Linked to Later Autism. http://www.unisci.com/stories/20012/0426011.htm

[6] Changeux, J., Danchin, A. (1976). Selective stabilization of developing synapses as a mechanism for the specification of neuronal networks. *Nature. Vol. 64*, No. 5588, pages 705-712.

[7] Eric Courchesne *et al.* (2007). Mapping Early Brain Development in Autism. *Neuron.Volume 56*, Issue 2, Pages 399-413.

[8] Nam J-K, Chung J-W, Kho H-S, Chung S-C, *et al.* (2007). Nerve growth factor concentration in human saliva. *Oral Disease, Volume 13*, Number 2, pages 187-192.

[9] Gehan A. Mostafa, Rasha T. Hamza, et al. (2008). Allergic manifestations in autistic children: Relation to disease Severity. *Journal of Pediatric Neurology. Volume 6*, Number 2, pages 115-123.

[10] Ballew Kinnaman. A brief natural history of rubber latex allergy. http://www.immune.com/rubber/nr1.html

[11] F. Edward Yazbal. Autism 2000. A Tragedy. http://www.whale.to/vaccine/ yazbak4.html

[12] Dan Olmsted. The Age of Autism, Science News. The Age of Autism, The Amish anomaly. http://www.upi.com/Science_News/2005/04/19/The-Age-of-Autism-The-Amish-anomaly/UPI-95661113911795/

[13] David G. Marsh, John D. Neely, Daniel R. Breazeale, *et al.* (1994). Linkage Analysis of IL4 and Other Chromosome 5q31.1 Markers and Total Serum Immunoglobulin E Concentrations. *Science.* pages 1152-1156.

[14] Herz U, Joachim R, Ahrens B, Scheffold A, *et al.* 2001). Allergic Sensitization and Allergen Exposure During Pregnancy Favor the Development of Atopy in the Neonate. *Int Arch Allergy Immunol. Vol. 124 (1-3)*, pages 193-196.

[15] Deborah Rice, Stan Barone Jr. (2000). Critical Periods of Vulnerability for the Developing Nervous System: Evidence from Humans and Animal Models. *Environmental Health Perspectives Supplements. Volume 108*, number S3.

[16] ABC News Online, Study links Autism and mother's illnesses, Tuesday, February 8, 2005, http://www.abc.net.au/news/newsitems/200502/ s1298671.htm.

[17] BE Mendyka, JM Clochesy, ML Workman, *et al.* Latex hypersensitivity: an iatrogenic and occupational risk. *American Journal of Critical care. Volume 3*, Issue 3, pages 198-201.

[18] Nancy A. Mitchell: Latex Allergy. Litigation. http://www.latexallergy links.org/lit.html

[19] Niggemann B, Kulig M, Bergmann R, *et al.* (1998). Development of latex allergy in children up to 5 years of age, a retrospective analysis of risk factors; Pedatr. *Allergy Immunol. Vol. 9*, No. 1, pages 36-39.

[20] Downing J. Dermatits from rubber gloves. *N England Journal of Medicine*, 1933; 208:196-8.

[21] Hans Asperger - Wikipedia, The free Encyclopedia. http://en.wikipedia. org/wiki/Hans_Asperger

[22] Ann G. Miguel, Glen R. Cass, Jay Weiss, et al. (1996). Latex Allergens in Tire Dust and Airborne Particles. *Environmental Health Perspectives. Volume 104*, No. 11.

[23] Michael R. Woolhiser, Albert E. Munson and B. Jean Meade. (2000). Immunological Responses of Mice following Administration of Natural Rubber Latex Proteins by Different Routes of Exposure. *Toxicological Sciences. Vol. 55*, pages 343-351.

[24] Harold D. Foster. (1999). Schizophrenia: The Latex Allergy Hypothesis. *Journal of Orthomolecular Medicine. Vol. 14*, No. 2, pages 83-90.

[25] Robin Mckie. (2001). Schizophrenia 'helped the ascent of man'. http://www.guardian.co.uk/Archive/Article/0,4273,4154224,00.html

Chapter V

THEORETICAL MODEL

As knowledge grows science must increasingly become the stimulus to imagination. – Edward O. Wilson

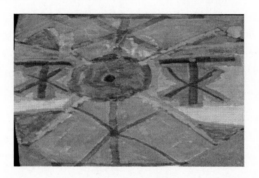

In the kindergarten year, Dain's autistic play activities were often directed at toy cars and toy trains. He placed the many colorful toys in a continuous line which stretched from room to room. The displacement of any of the cars or trains by a sibling or classmate was immediately replaced by Dain to continue the link. The excitement of organizing and maintaining the line of toys seemed to be a driving motivation in that if the line of toys was completely dismantled and placed in a storage container, he showed no frustration or anxiety about it. Alternatively, if he was taken away from the line of toys which remained on the floor he became very agitated. At around the same age, another autistic repetitive-behavior emerged which can simply be described as Dain's number 9 pattern. On the side of a hill in the backyard he would shuffle his feet, in a very athletic and fluid motion, to form a self induced path that ultimately became a deep trench over time. Hours, days, weeks, months, and years of shuffling on the same path etched a permanent scar in the landscape. Each cycle through the path brought forth euphoria of flapping hands, excited screams, and laughter. When it rained he enjoyed being soaked in mud and during a drought his feet, legs, and sometimes his whole body was covered in an earthy dust.

IS IT BECOMING MORE EVIDENT THAT NATURAL-LATEX ALLERGIES FAIL TO SHOW ANY BENEFITS AS IT RELATES TO BRAIN DEVELOPMENT?

It has been suggested that there are no folk medicine treatments using natural-latex. In contrast, most lacticiferous plants have many folk medicine applications to improve health [1].

Natural-latex contains many allergenic proteins. The World Health Organization - International Union of Immunological Societies has assigned names to thirteen of these allergens designated *Hev-b* 1 through *Hev-b* 13. There has been much research on the molecular structure of the *Hev-b* proteins. Immune responses to the *Hev-b* proteins and theoretical models of their relationship to allergy induced Autism is described below.

Hev-b 1

The *Hev-b* 1 protein (rubber elongation factor) has been shown to have HLA-DR4Dw4 (DRB1*040)-binding motif [2]. A *Hev-b* 1 immune response may induce Human leukocyte antigen recognition based on epitope homology. A study has shown that abnormal HLA-DR expression may affect the developing central nervous system during the second and third trimester [3].

Hev-b 2, Hev-b 7, and Hev-b 13

The *Hev-b* 2, *Hev-b* 7, and *Hev-b* 13 proteins (Lipolytic esterases) have been shown to have carbohydrate epitopes that may induce an immunoglobulin-E response [4,5]. A cross reaction to homologous glycoprotein may affect some of the symptoms of allergy induced Autism. As an example, maltase is an endogenous glycoprotein that breaks down maltose to glucose in the small intestine. Lower maltase activity has been associated with gastrointestinal dysfunction in some autistic children [6].

Furthermore, a study has shown that autoimmunity to brain proteins could play an etiopathogenic role in a subgroup of autistic patients. The frequency of serum anti-myelin—associated glycoprotein antibodies, as an index for autoimmunity to brain proteins, and their relation to family history of autoimmunity were investigated in 32 autistic and 32 healthy matched children. Autistic children had significantly higher serum anti-myelin—associated glycoprotein antibodies than healthy children (2100 [1995] and 1138 [87.5] Buhlmann titre unit, $P < .001$). Anti-myelin—associated glycoprotein positivity was elicited in 62.5 percent of autistic children. Family history of autoimmunity in autistic children (50%) was significantly higher than controls (9.4 percent). Anti-myelin—associated glycoprotein serum levels were significantly higher in autistic children with than those without such history ($P < .05$). In conclusion, Autism could be, in part, one of the pediatric autoimmune neuropsychiatric disorders. Further studies are warranted to shed light on the etiopathogenic role of anti-myelin—associated glycoprotein antibodies and the role of immunotherapy in Autism [7].

Hev-b 5

A study has indicated that about 75 percent of those on the Autism Spectrum are classified as mentally retarded [8]. *Hev-b* 5 (acidic latex protein) has high proline content of about14 percent to provide a tertiary structure having randoteric factors, inducing antibody recognition [9].

An endogenous protein that is known to greatly affect neuro-cognition is Fragile X m coil arrangement. Such an arrangement may inhibit enzymatic degradation, due to fragile X Mental Retardation Protein (FMRP). FMRP inhibition through a *Hev-b* cross-react immune response may play a direct role in the neural maturation process during prenatal/neonatal/infant development. For example, an immune response to the *Hev-b* 5 protein may affect glutamate expression. FMRP inhibition by glutamate disruption has been shown to affect the body's ability to translate mRNA [10].

In continuation, an acquired immune response to the *Hev-b* 5 protein may affect glutamic acid expression. Glutamic acid is the most abundant excitatory neurotransmitter and is involved in cognitive functions like learning and memory in the brain. Organisms synthesize gamma-aminobutyric acid (GABA) from glutamic acid. GABA disruption may affect prenatal Purkinje cell activity and formation. It is suspected that glutamate receptors and Shank3 proteins play a synergistic role in the density and maturation of elongated spines [11]. A secondary cooperative effect may exist between glutamate receptor activity and Shank3 during maturation of a nascent spine in a feed forward mechanism. Therefore, disruption of the glutamate/Shank3 mechanism may induce the formation of low-density and immature elongated spines often associated with mental retardation.

Hev-b 6

CD23 (or Fc epsilon RII) is a C-type lectin that functions as a receptor for immunoglobulin-E and is found on mature B-cells. In parallel, *Hev-b* 6 protein is a lectin-like protein that is a dominant allergen in Hevea brasiliensis natural-latex [12]. A *Hev-b* 6 protein (Hevein) induced immune response may affect the expression of CD23 on mature B-cells, affecting the regulation of immunoglobulin-E.

Hev-b 8

An immune-response to proteins homologous to *Hev-b* 8 protein may affect dendritic spine morphology. Profilin from mammalian cells is known to be a homologous protein to *Hev-b* 8 [13]. A *Hev-b* 8 protein (latex profilin) induced cross-react immune response to human profilin I, and to a lesser extent profilin II, may affect actin dynamics in synaptic plasticity [14].

Hev-b 9

Enolases are enzymes that participate in glycolysis by assisting in the conversion of glucose to pyruvate. *Hev-b* 9 displays an overall identity of 72 percent to human beta enolase [15]. A *Hev-b* 9 protein (latex enolase) induced cross-react immune response to human enolase may affect pyruvate levels through enzyme inhibition. Pyruvate deficiency has been associated with seizure and epilepsy. A study indicates that epilepsy in Autism Spectrum Disorders is a comorbid complication at rates of up to 33 percent [16]. Furthermore, a *Hev-b* 9 induced cross-react immune response to exogenous enolases (e.g., yeast infection) may further affect allergy induced Autism. It is well known that homologous enolases from yeasts, molds, and fungi are known to cross-react with *Hev-b* 9 [17,18]. A study indicates that elevated levels of Candida Albicans in some autistic individuals may exacerbate many behavior and health problems, especially those with late-onset Autism [19]. Thus, enolase over-expression and subsequent immune sensitivity may trigger hyper adaptive-immunity affecting the atypicality of allergy induced Autism.

Hev-b 10

Superoxide dismutase is a potential cross-react protein associated with a *Hev-b* 10 immune response. Superoxide dismutase enzymes such as magnesium Superoxide dismutase are important antioxidant-defense proteins in nearly all cells exposed to oxygen. A study has shown that cross-reactive allergens play an increasingly important role in latex allergy in complicating both the diagnosis and time course of allergic symptoms. Manganese superoxide dismutase, a ubiquitous protein of prokaryotic and eukaryotic organisms, was described as a cross-reactive allergen in Aspergillus fumigatus. Little information is available on the importance of this pan-allergen in Hevea brasiliensis latex. The aim of this study was to clone and express manganese superoxide dismutase from H. brasiliensis latex, and to obtain the soluble and immunologically active recombinant allergen for diagnosis of latex allergy and to investigate possible cross-reactivities with the structurally related A. fumigatus and human manganese superoxide dismutase. The research concluded that Hev b 10 is a new cross-reactive allergen of Hevea brasiliensis which belongs to the 'latex-mold' group of latex allergens. Furthermore, it is a candidate for primary sensitization in patients allergic to the pan-allergen manganese superoxide dismutase [20]. Another study has shown that antioxidant enzyme activities may play a role in the pathophysiological mechanisms involved in Autism [21].

Hev-b 11

Hevea brasiliensis natural-latex contains high levels of both chitinases and lysozymes [22]. Human chitotriosidase is a potential cross-react protein associated with a *Hev-b* 11 protein immune response based on its homology to the chitinase family of proteins [23]. A *Hev-b* 11 protein (class I endochitinase) induced cross-react immune response to human chitotriosidase and plant-based chitinase may affect fungal immunity and food allergies in allergy induced Autism. It has been shown that chitotriosidase deficiency may play a role in digestion of chitin-containing food as well as defense against chitin-coated microorganisms and parasites [24,25].

If Regressive Autism is influenced by allergic responses during prenatal/neonatal/infant development, then later onset of such an acquired immune response may affect neuro-cognitive development in older children. For example, attention-deficit hyperactivity disorder often occurs in children between the ages of three to seven. In speculation, acquired allergies and cross-react immune responses at this period of brain development may affect the atypicality of attention-deficit hyperactivity disorders (A.D.H.D.).

Does Immune Sensitivity to the Allergens in Natural-Latex Affect Learning and Intelligence?

Immune responses to the allergenic proteins in natural-latex may also be affecting neuro-cognitive development in individuals with spina bifida/hydrocephalus. Studies have shown that about 73 percent of individuals with spina bifida/hydrocephalus have natural-latex allergy. Increased sensitization in this population is related to early, frequent exposure to natural-latex products such as catheters used in bladder programs. These children also tend to have frequent surgeries and diagnostic tests, which increases their exposure to natural-latex gloves. There is a broad range of scores on intelligence tests among children with spina bifida/hydrocephalus ranging from the gifted to the retarded. It is generally recognized that learning problems are routinely a part of children with spina bifida/hydrocephalus including attention, perceptual motor processes, reasoning and problem solving, organization and sequencing skills, and memory [26,27].

Natural-latex allergies affect development, and it is becoming more evident that such allergies fail to show any benefits as it relates to child development. Therefore, we must ask ourselves should extreme measures be taken to reduce exposure. Some of the most potentially gifted and talented individuals have been irreversibly damaged from over-exposure to the allergenic proteins in natural-latex.

REFERENCES

[1] James A. Duke. Hevea brasiliensis (Willd.) Muell.-Arg, 1983 Handbook of the Energy Corps. http://www.hort.purdue.edu/newcrop/duke_energy/Hevea_ brasiliensis.html#Folk%20Medicine

[2] Raulf-Heimsoth M, Chen Z, Rihs HP, Kalbacher H, Liebers V, et al. (1998). Analysis of T-cell reactive regions and HLA-DR4 binding motifs on the latex allergen Hev b 1 (rubber elongation factor). Clin Exp Allergy. Vol. 28, No. 3, pages 339-48.

[3] Wierzba-Bobrowicz T, Kosno-Kruszewska E, Gwiazda E, et al. (2000). Major histocompatability complex class II (MHC II) expression during the development of human fetal cerebral occipital lobe, cerebellum, and hematopoietic organs. Folia Neuropathol. Vol. 38, pages 111–118.

[4] Yagami T, Osuna H, Kouno M, et al. (2002). Significance of carbohydrate epitopes in a latex allergen with beta-1, 3-glucanase activity. Int. Arch Allergy Immunol. Vol.129. No. 1, pages 27-37.

[5] Siti Arija M. Arif, Robert G. Hamilton, Faridah Yusof, et al. (2004). Isolation and Characterization of the Early Nodule-specific Protein Homologue (Hev b 13), an Allergenic Lipolytic Esterase from Hevea brasiliensis Latex; J. Biol. Chem., Vol. 279, Issue 23, pages 23933-23941.

[6] Rafail Kushak, Harland Winter, Nathan Farber, et al. (2005). Gastrointestinal symptoms and intestinal disaccharides activities in children with Autism. Journal of Pediatric Gastroenterology and Nutrition. Vol. 41, No. 4.

[7] Zeinab Awad El-Sayed, Manal Mohamed Abd El-Aziz, Mohamed Farouk El-Sayed. (2008). Serum Anti-Myelin—Associated Glycoprotein Anti bodies in Egyptian Autistic Children. Journal of Child Neurology, Volume 23, Number 12, pages 1413-1418

[8] CDM van Karnebeek et al. (2002). An aetiological study of 25 mentally retarded adults with Autism. Journal of Medical Genetics. Vol. 39, pages 205-213.

[9] Jay E. Slater, Thomas Vedvick, Ann Arther-Smith, *et al.* (1996). Identification, Cloning, and Sequence of a Major Allergen (Hev b 5) from Natural Rubber Latex (Hevea brasiliensis). *The Journal of Biological Chemistry. Vol. 271*, No. 41, pages 25391-25399.

[10] William T. Greenough, Anna Y. Klintsova, Scott A. Irwin, *et al.* (2001). Synaptic regulation of protein synthesis and the fragile X protein. *Proc Natl Acad Sci U S A. Vol. 98*, No. 13, pages 7101–7106.

[11] Gautier Roussignol, Fabrice Ango, Stefano Romorini, et al. (2005). Shank Expression Is Sufficient to Induce Functional Dendrite Spine Synapses in Aspiny Neurons. *The Journal of Neuroscience. Vol. 25*, No. 14, pages 3560-3570.

[12] Gidrol X., Chrestin H., Tan HuiLang, *et al.* (1994). Hevein, a lectin-like protein from Hevea brasiliensis (rubber tree) is involved in the coagulation of latex. *Journal of Biological Chemistry. Vol. 269*, No. 12, pages 9278-9283.

[13] Matthew B. Mellon, Brendon T. Frank, Kenneth C. Fang. (2002). Mast Cell -Chymase Reduces IgE Recognition of Birch Pollen Profilin by Cleaving Antibody-Binding Epitopes. *The Journal of Immunology. Vol. 168*, pages 290-297.

[14] Manuel Ackermann, Andrew Matus. (2003). Activity-induced targeting of profilin and stabilization of dendritic spine morphology. *Nature Neuroscience. Vol. 6*, No. 11, pages 1194-1200.

[15] Wagner et al. (2000). Hev b 9, an enolase and a new cross-react allergen from Hevea latex and molds. *Eur. J. Biochem. Vol. 267*, pages 7006-7014.

[16] Tuchman R, Rapin I. (2002). Epilepsy in Autism. *Lancet Neurology. Vol. 1*, pages 352-358.

[17] Wagner et al. (2000). Hev b 9, an enolase and a new cross-react allergen from Hevea latex and molds. *Eur. J. Biochem. Vol. 267*, pages 7006-7014.

[18] Ito K, Ishiguro A, Kanbe T, Tanaka K, Torii S. (1995). Detection of IgE antibody against candida albicans enolase and its cross-reactivity to sarcharomyes cerevisiae; *Clin Exp Allergy. Vol. 25*, No. 6, pages 522-8.

[19] Stephen M. Edelson: The Candida Yeast-Autism Connection; Center for the Study of Autism, Salem, Oregon. http://www.mold-survivor.com/candida_yeast.html

[20] Wagner S, Sowka S, Mayer C, *et al.* (2001). Identification of a Hevea brasiliensis latex manganese superoxide dismutase (Hev b 10) as a cross-reactive allergen. *Int Arch Allergy Immunol. Vol. 125*, pages120–127.

[21] Söüt S; Zorolu SS, Ozyurt H, Yilmaz HR, *et al.* (2003). Changes in nitric oxide levels and antioxidant enzyme activities may have a role in the pathophysiological mechanisms involved in Autism. *Clin Chim Acta. Vol. 331*, No 1-2, pages 111-117.

[22] Melinda N. Martin. (1991). The Latex of Hevea brasiliensis contains high levels of both chitinases and chitinases/lysozymes. *Plant Physiology. Vol. 95*, No. 2, pages 469-476.

[23] O'Riordain G, Radauer C, Hoffam-Sommergruber K, *et al.* (2002). Cloning and molecular characterization of the Hevea brasiliensis allergen *Hev-b* 11, a class I chitinases. *Clin, Exp. Allergy. Vol. 32*, No. 3, pages 455-62.

[24] Renkema GH, Boot RG, Muijsers AO, et al. (1995). Purification and characterization of Human chitotriosidase, a novel member of the chitinase family of proteins. *J. Bio. Chem., Vol. 270*, No. 5, pages 2198-202.

[25] Masaka S uzuki, Wakako Fujimoto, Marie Goto, *et al.* (2002). Cellular Expression of GutChitinase mRNA in Gastrointestinal Tract of Mice and Chickens. *Journal of Histochemical and Cytochemistry. Vol. 50*, pages 1081-1089.

[26] Kelly KI, Pearson ML, Kurup VP, *et al.* (1994). A cluster of anaphylactic reactions in spina bifida during general anesthesia. *J Allergy Clin Immunol. Vol. 94*, pages 53-61.

[27] Spina Bifida Association of America. http://www.spinabifidaassociation. org/site/c.liKWL7PLLrF/b.2642297/k.5F7C/Spina_Bifida_Association.htm

Chapter VI

GENDER

The gender difference in immunity guides our knowledge and strengthens our future. - Michael J. Dochniak

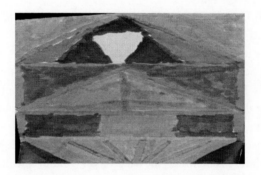

At the age of eleven, Dain had the communication skills of an infant but the physical attributes of a young adult - deep vocal pitch, fast growing facial hair, and unusual muscularity had prematurely turned this autistic boy into a young man. A pronounced physical strength and the inability to communicate his needs often resulted in self injurious behaviors. As an example, an automobile drive often initiated hand biting and head slapping in that his inability to perceive the purpose of the drive caused much anxiety and frustration. Using pictures as a visual clue of the destination failed to provide any relief for him. In the many twists and turns of Regressive Autism, for many years he often screamed on right turns. Occasionally, car trips were planned in such a way as to avoid an excess of right turns. Eventually, this behavior stopped abruptly with no indication for its disappearance.

Does the Expression of Hormones and Immunoglobulin-E Show that Males and Females have Different Immunity?

The ratio of gender within the Autism Spectrum is about 4:1 (male/female). Immunological differences based on gender may have affected the frequency and intensity of adaptive immune responses associated with allergy induced Autism. For example, it is known that the ratio of food allergies based on gender is about 2:1 (male/female). Furthermore, childhood asthma has also been shown to occur at about a 3:1 ratio (male/female), especially amongst young children.

Does Hormone Expression Affect the Incidence and Atypicality of Allergy Induced Autism?

A study has shown that sex differences exist in asthma and atopy with a preponderance of boys before puberty. There is a reversal of this sex ratio during puberty with girls having more asthma and atopy throughout the reproductive years. Elucidating the reasons for the switch in the sex ratio should provide fresh insights into asthma and atopy with a real prospect of novel therapies for these troublesome diseases. The challenge is to match the epidemiology and physiology with the accumulating scientific knowledge on gender differences in immune responses. Hormonal changes have been implicated in the reversal of the sex ratio. Testosterone is an immuno-suppressant and is likely to be protective, while female sex steroids are pro-inflammatory and will increase the susceptibility to atopy. The research showed that sex steroids could play a useful part in modulating the immunological and inflammatory processes that underlie asthma and other allergic disorders, complementing the currently used glucocorticoid derived steroids [1].

Furthermore, a study on the effects of gender on allergen-induced histamine release in ongoing allergic cutaneous reactions concluded gender does influence the degree of invivo antigen-induced histamine release from mast cells. The research showed that male subjects released higher amounts of histamine in the first hour than female subjects [2].

In animal studies, research on the differences in concentration of endogenous proteins in sex organs of BALB/c mice has shown that levels of neuron growth factor and immunoglobulin-E were consistently higher in organs of male mice in comparison to their female siblings [3].

Another theory on the incidence of Autism Spectrum Disorders and gender has been directed at testosterone which is the principle male sex hormone. Research suggests that there may be a link between Autism and testosterone levels in the womb as the fetus develops. For example, research from Cambridge University has shown that babies who produce high levels of testosterone while they are still in the womb have a higher chance of showing Autism Spectrum Disorder traits later on [4].

Thus, the immune system of males and females are different and it appears that the expression of hormones and immunoglobulin-E affects the gender incidence of allergy induced Autism.

REFERENCES

[1] M Osman. (2003). Therapeutic implications of sex differences in asthma and atopy, *Disease of Childhood.Vol. 88*, pages 587-590.

[2] Aikins PC, Von Allmen C, Valenzano M, *et al.* (1193). The effects of gender on allergen-induced histamine release in ongoing allergic cutaneous reactions. *J. Allergy Clin. Immunol. Vol. 91*, No. 5, pages 1031-1040.

[3] Binie V. Lipps (2002). Age and sex-related difference in levels of nerve growth factor in organs of BALB/c mice. *Journal of Natural Toxins. Vol. 11*, pages 387-391.

[4] Autism News. (2004). Autism and testosterone levels in the womb possible link. http://windowsupdatecenter.com/?id=198760218

Chapter VII

GENETICS

Genetics is crude, but neuroscience goes directly to work on the brain, and the mind follows. - Leon Kass

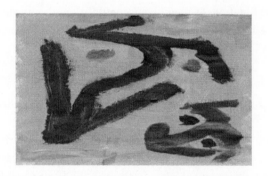

A large population of autistic children, including Dain and his sibling, were studied by the University of Iowa to determine if there were any genetic markers associated Autism Spectrum Disorders. The research showed that there were no definitive answers to a genetic etiology. Furthermore a medical review covering several generations showed that there was no incidence of Autism or mental retardation in Dain's family history. There is a genetic predisposition for humans to explore their surroundings and Dain was no exception. For safety reasons a six foot high fence, with locked gates, was constructed around his backyard. For many years, this proved to be an effective barrier keeping him safe inside. His first successful attempt to scale the fence and explore the mystery of the outside would be his last. Dragging a large plastic container up to the fence, he was able to escape without anyone noticing. Soon, his parents realized that he was gone and a frantic search ensued. Thirty minutes later a report came in that a young man had entered a house and rummaged through the refrigerator before leaving. Wandering further through the neighborhood, Dain was eventually located in a garage about 1/2-mile from his house. Bleeding and frustrated, he huddled in darkness biting his hand and scratching his cheeks. The first familiar face brought out a noticeable giggle and smile. Dain was safe but the world outside the fence had now become a confusing and scary place.

DOES THE SIMPLEST SOLUTION TEND TO BE THE BEST SOLUTION?

Learning and intelligence is often thought of as genetically influenced wherein the mind and body is pre-engineered (e.g., neurological development) to effectively gather, store, and retrieve chemical information. Many researchers suspect that a combination of genetic susceptibility and environmental insult are involved in the etiology of Autism Spectrum Disorders. Several examples of candidate gene loci are described below.

Chromosome 1 (1q23, Fc fragment of immunoglobulin-E)

As a part of the study of Autism Spectrum Disorders in the Finnish population, researchers performed an extensive genealogical search and identified common ancestors for a set of study families. They were able to connect 21 Finnish Autism families by genealogical links extending to 17th century. A genome-wide scan of 1100 micro-satellites yielding an average 4cM grid was performed in the 21 nuclear families (number of affected = 31) belonging to the pedigree. Joint analysis of linkage and linkage disequilibrium (LD) was performed by using Pseudo-marker statistics. The best evidence for joint linkage and LD emerged for loci at 1q23 (p=0.0008). The 1q23 locus has been among the best loci also in the two earlier genome-wide scans in the Finnish sample (Auranen et al. 2002; Ylisaukko-oja et al. 2004). Next, they performed fine mapping of the identified loci by using dense set of micro satellites as well as SNPs at several positional candidates including e.g. RGS4 and NOS1AP at 1q23 as well as GABA receptor cluster at 15q12. The best association evidence was observed at 1q23, in which one of the intragenic SNPs yielded p=0.0001 in the Pseudo-marker analysis. This result was further supported by suggestive association evidence at the flanking SNPs [1].

Chromosome 11 (11q12-q13, immunoglobulin-E Responsiveness)

Research has described the chromosomal localization of the gene for squamous cell carcinoma-associated reactive antigen for cytotoxic T cells (SART-1). The *SART-1* gene localized to a region of 11q12–13 showing strong linkage to atopy in previous studies. Further analysis of this gene revealed the presence of at least 20 exons of varying lengths and four novel single-nucleotide polymorphisms, one of which resulted in an amino acid substitution. Association analysis in families recruited on the basis of affected sib pairs for asthma reveal significant association for both coding region polymorphisms with atopy. We therefore hypothesize that polymorphic variation within the *SART-1* gene may account for individuals developing atopy [2].

Chromosome 19 (19p13.3, CD23)

Research has demonstrated the role of a proteolytic enzyme called ADAM10 that releases a major allergy regulatory protein from the surface of cells and thereby promotes a stronger allergic response. The identification of drugs that inhibit ADAM10's ability to release this molecule could revolutionize treatment of asthma and allergic disease. The research showed that allergic disease can be modulated by high levels of the regulatory protein, known as CD23, which ultimately results in a decreased production of immunoglobulin-E. The research also showed that when the regulatory protein is released from the cell surface by ADAM10 there is an increase in the production of immunoglobulin-E and therefore, increased allergy [3].

Chromosome X (Xp11.23, FOXP3)

Research has shown that the forkhead-winged helix family transcription factor, *Foxp3*, has been shown to be specifically expressed in murine $CD25^+CD4^+$ T_R cells and as such appears to be a 'master gene' controlling the development and suppressive function of these cells. Thus $CD4^+CD25^+$ T_R cells constitute a functionally and developmentally unique subpopulation of T cells [4].

Furthermore, allergy induced Autism may involve environmentally induced epigenetic mechanisms. It's generally recognized that epigenetic mechanisms may influence cytokine gene expression in a naive CD4+ T cell as it develops into a Th1 or Th2 cell [5].

Is the Etiology of Autism Spectrum Disorders based on a Precondition of Atopy and Increased Environmental Insult?

The concept of Occam's razor is often paraphrased, *all things being equal; the simplest solution tends to be the best one.* Using this concept, one may decide which statement or combinations of statements encompass the spirit of Occam's razor and Autism Spectrum Disorders:

The increased incidence of Autism Spectrum Disorders is influenced by a global increase of genetic mutations resulting in atypical protein transcription/expression;

The increased incidence of Autism Spectrum Disorders is influenced by a global increase of epigenetic mechanisms resulting in atypical protein transcription/expression; and

The increased incidence of Autism Spectrum Disorders is influenced by a global increase of allergies resulting in atypical protein transcription/expression.

REFERENCES

[1]   Tero Ylisaukko-oja, Helena Kilpinen, Reija Alen, *et al.* (2006). Genome-wide Scan for Autism in an Extended Pedigree from a Regional Subisolate in Finland. *Hugo's 11th Human Genome Meeting, Helsinki Fair Centre, Helsinki Finland, Workshop 3*, Poster 45.

[2]   Amanda P. Wheatley, Daniel J. Bollard, Jane E. et al. (2002). Identification of the development of atopy. *Human Molecular Genetics. Vol. 11*, No. 18, pages 2143-2146.

[3]   Medical News Today. Key Molecular Signaling Switch Involved In Allergic Disease Identification. http://www.medicalnewstoday.com/articles/ 55360. php

[4] Zoltan Fehervari, Shimon Sakaguchi. (2004). Control of Foxp3+ CD25+ CD4+ regulating cell activation and function by dendritic cells. *International Immunology. Vol. 16*, No. 12, pages 1769-1780.

[5] Virginia M. Sanders. (2005). Epigenetic Regulation of Th1 and Th2 Cell development. *Brain, Behavior, and Immunity. August 6*, 2005, ELSEVIER.

Chapter VIII

COMORBIDITY

Science is the desire to know causes. -William Hazlitt

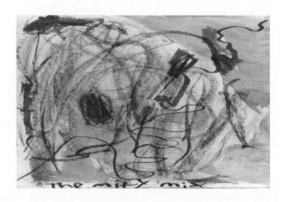

With intense focus and precision, Dain would skillfully empty and fill containers with different types of liquids and solids. Water, milk, maple syrup, fruit juices, bread, vegetables and other foodstuff items were combined into cups and glasses to provide a miraculously measured culinary-mess. Another activity that held Dain's focus in his early teens revolved around watching videos. Fast forwarding and rewinding videos at specific locations provided much needed stimulation for him. Occasionally, if a car or *Thomas the Tank* train in the video went off screen he would climb on the television in an attempt to locate it. This eventually destroyed hundreds of video cassettes, dozen of video cassette players, and a few televisions before the behavior wore itself out.

Is the Cause of Autism
the Ultimate Challenge?

It has been speculated that television is involved in the etiology of Autism Spectrum Disorders. A Cornell University economics professor and associates have written a research paper suggesting that scientists study the connection between early childhood television viewing and Autism. Their basic thesis: Excessive TV viewing by children with a genetic disposition to Autism makes them more likely to develop the disorder [1]. Is visual over-stimulation a comorbid factor in the etiology of allergy induced Autism?

There are often comorbid factors that affect the atypicality of Autism Spectrum Disorders. The term "comorbid" often has two meanings: to indicate a medical condition existing simultaneously but independently with another condition in a person; and to indicate a medical condition in a person that causes, is caused by, or is otherwise related to another condition in the same person.

Comorbid interactions that may be associated with the etiology of allergy induced Autism include the following:

Infection

Infection and natural-latex sensitivity may be a comorbid factor.

A study published in *Pediatrics* investigated the association between infections in the first 2 years and subsequent diagnosis of Autism Spectrum Disorders. The research showed that children with subsequent diagnosis of Autism do not have more overall infections in the first 2 years of life than children without Autism [2].

It is well known that allergies are often prevalent in children with Autism Spectrum Disorders [3]. A combination of infection and environmental insult may affect the development of allergies. For example, Johns Hopkins scientists have found the first hard evidence that viral infections can induce asthma and allergies, a connection long suspected but never directly confirmed in the lab. They showed that weak viral infections can cause immune system B-cells to produce immunoglobulin E, a protein that orchestrates the reactions that cause allergies [4].

Furthermore, it has been shown that prenatal and early postnatal environments are significant predictors of total immunoglobulin concentration in adolescents. The research showed that infectious disease in infancy, as well as interactions between prenatal and postnatal environments, appear to have long-term effects on adolescent total immunoglobulin-E production [5].

An example wherein a stealth chronic-infection may be a comorbid factor in the cause of allergy induced Autism is Lyme disease. An epidemiologic study is evaluating if there is a connection to the prevalence of Lyme disease and Autism in children.

Infection may also induce autoimmunity when atopy is present. Specifically, infectious agents may cause mammalian cells to release endogenous protein-fragments that can induce an immune response. Briefly, in the formation of endogenous-proteins deoxyribonucleic acid (DNA) is transcribed in the cells nucleus into messenger ribonucleic acid (mRNA). The mRNA is then exported to the cytoplasm for translation into protein. Translation occurs in ribosome's wherein transfer RNA (tRNA) deliver amino acids which are then bonded together to form a protein chain. During an infection (e.g., viral), propagation within the cell can rupture the cell wall. Once cell containment is breached, tRNA-based protein-fragments within the cytoplasm can then leach into circulation through diffusion. When atopy is present, the increased prevalence of b-cells (i.e., plasma & memory) and the fragments incomplete structure (e.g., nucleoprotein fragments) may induce an immune response. An immune response to the protein fragment may increase the probability of a cross-react immune response to endogenous proteins having a homologous protein-fragment therein. Because different cells produce different proteins, the type of cell infected may induce autoimmunity based on the cells genetic information.

Chronic infection and/or dampened immunity may affect the gender incidence of allergy induced Autism. As previously discussed, studies have shown that increased testosterone levels tend to blunt innate immunity affecting the prevalence of infection. The comorbid interaction of infections, allergies, and testosterone expression may help explain the 4:1 (male/female) gender incidence of Autism Spectrum Disorders.

Vaccines

Vaccinations and natural-latex sensitivity may be a comorbid factor.

Much attention has been given to the theory that vaccinations may have increased the incidence of Autism Spectrum Disorders. For example, it has been proposed that the mercurial-based preservative (i.e., Thimerosal) in vaccines cause adverse neurological development, and other biochemical disruptions, that may increase the incidence of Autism Spectrum Disorders. Although mercury-based organics are well known to be harmful to the central nervous system in all individuals, its role in the development of Autism Spectrum Disorders continues to be debated.

The Measles, Mumps, and Rubella vaccine has also been suspected in the cause of Autism Spectrum Disorders. Vaccines are a preparation of killed microorganisms, or living attenuated organisms, or living fully virulent organisms that are administered to produce or artificially increase immunity to a particular disease. The microorganisms in the vaccines are composed of exogenous proteins that can inherently trigger an immune response. Furthermore, other protein additives in the vaccines have been shown to cause allergic reactions. Studies have shown that the presence of gelatin in the Measles, Mumps, and Rubella vaccine may intensify the immune response in atopic individuals [6].

Oxytocin

Oxytocin and natural-latex sensitivity may be a comorbid factor.

Oxytocin is a mammalian hormone that acts as a neurotransmitter in the brain. A study on the role of Oxytocin in natural-latex allergy during Cesarean-Section showed the vaso-and utero constrictor effects of administered Oxytocin worsened the expression of natural-latex allergy [7].

Administered Oxytocin during the birthing process may have increased the incidence of prenatal/neonatal/infant natural-latex allergy during the birthing process. The structure of Oxytocin shows similar homology to endogenous epitopes to some of the allergenic proteins in natural-latex based on the presence of cysteine residues that form a sulfur bridge.

Fever

Postoperative fever and natural-latex sensitivity may be a comorbid factor.

Increased body temperature and blood flow has been shown to affect the binding rates of antibodies and allergens. For example, leukocytes are known to display a "shear threshold effect"; this effect is due to an increase in collisions between receptor and ligand with increasing shear [8].

Collision theory of reaction rates associated with adaptive immunity is important in guiding our understanding of allergy induced Autism. Several factors that may affect the frequency and intensity of the adaptive immune response include: the quantity of allergenic proteins in a unit volume of blood; prevalence of somatic hyper-mutation or affinity maturation of lymphocytes specific to the allergenic protein in a unit volume of blood; and increased body temperature and blood flow.

Gut Microflora

Gut micro-flora and natural-latex sensitivity may be a comorbid factor.

A study that explored allergy development and the intestinal micro-flora during the first year of life concluded that differences in the composition of the gut flora between infants who will and infants who will not develop allergy are demonstrable before the development of any clinical manifestations of atopy [9].

In a theoretical model, a natural-latex induced immune-response during neonatal development may affect some of the symptoms of allergy induced Autism through atypical micro-flora expression. For example, the cell wall of gram positive bacteria is primarily composed of peptidoglycans, approximately 90 percent. Peptidoglycans are polymers that consist of sugars and amino acids. A natural-latex immune response (e.g., *Hev-b* 2, *Hev-b* 7, *Hev-b* 13) may induce cross reactivity to some gram positive bacteria including enterococci and bifidobacteria based on carbohydrate epitopes (e.g., n-acetyglucosamine), affecting the incidence and prevalence of hyper adaptive immunity. It is recognized that one of the potential symptoms of natural-latex sensitivity is diarrhea.

Sleep

Sleep and natural-latex sensitivity may be a comorbid factor.

During an allergic response, immunoglobulin-E primed mast-cells bind to the allergen and release the neurotransmitter histamine through a process called degranulation. Histamine expression affects wakefulness; it has been shown that histaminergic cells have the most wakefulness-related firing pattern of any neuronal type thus far recorded.

In continuation, it is known that young children with Autism Spectrum Disorders often have sleep difficulties [10]. In other sleep studies, histamine has been implicated as a significant endogenous compound involved with wakefulness [11,12].

Active sleep is particularly important to the developing brain, possibly because it provides the neural stimulation that newborns need to form mature neural connections and for proper nervous system development. Studies investigating the effects of active sleep deprivation have shown that deprivation early in life can result in behavioral problems, permanent sleep disruption, decreased brain mass, and result in an abnormal amount of neuronal cell death. Rapid eye movement (REM) sleep is necessary for proper central nervous system development. Thus, natural-latex sensitivity affects histamine expression; inducing irregular patterns of active sleep during child development.

Immunoglobulin-E

Immunoglobulin-E expression and natural-latex sensitivity may be a comorbid factor.

A study has shown that seventy five percent of people with natural-latex allergy are female and this is possibly due to a higher proportion of women in the exposed population. Additional exposure risks may arise from: obstetric procedures; gynecological examinations; contact with contraceptives; and certain professions like doctors, nurses, scientists which carry an increased risk of occupational exposure Hevea brasiliensis natural-latex [13].

The prevalence of an IgE antibody induced immune response during pregnancy may affect the intra uterine environment. The atopic history of parents has long been used to predict infant atopy. Research has shown that maternal, but not paternal, total immunoglobulin-E level correlates with elevated infant immunoglobulin-E levels and infant atopy; which suggests that maternal factor, placental factors, or both have an impact on perinatal allergic sensitization [14]. In parallel, another study indicates that parental immunoglobulin-E levels may be an indicator of atopy in young children and the study showed that boys have higher immunoglobulin-E levels compared to girls [15].

During neonatal development, the kinetics and courses of allergen-specific antibody responses suggest that, once established, allergen-specific immunoglobulin-E responses are driven by antigen contact rather than cytokines controlling class switch to immunoglobulin-E [16].

Research has shown that some dendritic cells, as well as mast cells and basophils, express the high affinity receptor for immunoglobulin-E (Fc epsilon R1). This finding has important implications since dendritic cells play an important role in antigen presentation to T lymphocytes. If immunoglobulin-E antibodies present in atopic individuals bind to such Fc epsilon R1 on dendritic cells, subsequent exposure of such dendritic cells to the offending allergen may enhance presentation of epitopes in such allergens to T cells, further enhancing the allergic immune response. The authors concluded that the serum immunoglobulin-E is a major factor driving Fc epsilon R1 expression on dendritic cells [17].

Cysteine-rich Proteins

Protein insult and natural-latex sensitivity maybe a comorbid factor.

The cysteine residues in natural-latex proteins have been shown to play a major role in allergenicity. Research has shown that recombinant natural-latex allergens wherein the cysteine residues are replaced with alanine form peptide variants that have markedly decreased immunoglobulin-E binding. Furthermore, basophile activation testing has shown decreased activation with successive cysteine exclusion [18].

Examples of an adaptive immune response to cysteine-rich proteins include proteases which are often used as food additives and function as digestive enzymes. The proteases papain and bromelain, which are homologous proteins to some of the *Hev-b* proteins, can cause allergic reactions in individuals having a natural-latex allergy.

In a theoretical model, an acquired immune response to natural-latex may affect the methionine pathway and P450 detoxification system through a cross-react immune response based on primary and/or tertiary structure homology. The expressions of other cysteine-rich endogenous proteins have been implicated in Autism Spectrum Disorders including Metallothionein proteins [19].

Prostaglandins

Prostaglandin expression and natural-latex sensitivity may be a comorbid factor.

Natural-latex cause IgE primed mast cells and basophils to release inflammatory agents which may affect the expression of touch allodynia. As an example, during prenatal development maternal immune responses to allergens are known to increase the expression of prostaglandins [20]. A study indicates that the balance of prostaglandin D2 (PGD2) and prostaglandin E2 (PGE2) may play a role in innocuous tactile stimuli evoked pain [21].

Touch allodynia has also been observed to be a symptom for some Autistic individual's. Touch allodynia is an exaggerated response to a non-noxious stimulus and can be either static or mechanical. A person with touch allodynia may perceive light pressure or the movement of clothes over the skin as painful, whereas a "normal" individual will not feel pain

Endorphins

Endorphin expression and natural-latex sensitivity may be a comorbid factor.

Endorphins are endogenous opioid neuro-peptides that are considered "natural pain killers". A study has shown that circulating leukocytes can synthesize, store, and release endorphins. The research showed that there is increasing evidence for a bidirectional communications system between the immune system and the brain. Many of the substances involved in this communication appear to be neuro-peptides. These findings have given biochemical validity to the clinical and epidemiological studies that have suggested that psychosocial factors can modulate the response to infections and neoplasm's [22].

The recent finding of nerve growth factor in mast cells widens the spectrum of potential responses that back-fed peripheral neurons can produce during neuro-immune interactions. Also, nerve growth factor has been shown to govern the enhanced ability of endorphins to suppress inflammatory pain [23]. Thus, the frequency and intensity of an acquired immune response to the proteins in natural-latex may induce endorphin and neuron growth factor over-expression to affect some of the symptoms of allergy induced Autism.

Amino Acids

Amino acid expression and natural-latex sensitivity may be a comorbid factor.

A cross-react immune response to nutritional food-stuff proteins may affect the body's protein-cycle resulting in amino acid imbalance. Foodstuff proteins are often broken down into amino acids that are used as building blocks to make other proteins essential for life. There are certain amino acids that are classified as "essential" meaning they must be attained from foodstuff proteins. Tryptophan is an essential amino acid that serves as a precursor for the neurotransmitter serotonin.

Food allergies induced by natural-latex may affect the expression of essential amino acids such as Methionine and Tryptophan that are used to produce neurotransmitters. A study examined serotonergic and noradrenergic markers and found that plasma concentrations of tryptophan, the precursor of serotonin, were significantly lower in autistic patients than in healthy volunteers. Research has shown that lowered plasma tryptophan may play a role in the pathophysiology of Autism [24].

Furthermore, the protein cycle is further stressed to accommodate immunoglobulin-E and mast cell proliferation and/or replacement. Thus, the frequency and intensity of food allergies induced by natural-latex may adversely affect the expression of amino acid during critical stages of brain development.

Blood Type

Blood type and natural-latex sensitivity may be a comorbid factor.

Although there is not a published study, an informal accounting shows a marked prevalence of blood type-A among autistic children. The other blood types generally appear to have low incidence, risk or severity of Autism Spectrum Disorders.

The allergenic protein Hev-6 is a lectin-type protein. Lectins are known to play important roles in the immune system by recognizing carbohydrates. Lectins are a type of receptor protein that recognizes and bind to monosaccharides including N-acetyglucosamine and N-acetygalactosamine. Unlike other blood types, blood type-A contains extra N-acetylgalactosamine. In a theoretical model, blood type A associated with a *Hev-b* 6 induced immune response may affect the trimerization of immunoglobulin-E primed mast cells (i.e., degranulation) based on structure homology.

The Para rubber tree initially grew in South America where it was the main source of natural-latex consumed during the 19th century. Also, the Mayan's of Central America have a long history of rubber usage. Hundreds of years of *Hev-b* protein exposure have not appeared to have dramatically affected Autism Spectrum Disorders in these cultures. Blood type may have protected them in that Native South American's have 100 percent of the blood type-O and 98 percent of the Mayan population has the blood type-O.

Allergenic rubber-proteins may have stressed adaptive immune systems throughout history independent of blood type. Modern evidence has shown that the Mesoamericans including the Maya and Aztec, who had some of the most complex and advanced cultures, exploited stabilized natural rubber from the lacticiferous plant Castilla elastica as early as 1600 before Christ (B.C.).

Did stressed adaptive-immunity from rubber allergens affect the incidence of cognitive atypicality wherein some cases may have been perceived as "psychological disorders"?

Did a misunderstanding and fear of such cognitive atypicality lead to a path of great violence and destruction, e.g., ritualistic human sacrifices to their Gods?

In parallel, the increased incidence of allergy induced Autism in industrialized societies worldwide continues to present the ultimate challenge.

Neurotransmitters

Neurotransmitter expression and natural-latex sensitivity may be a comorbid factor.

A study has shown that one of the most consistent biological findings in Autism is elevated blood serotonin levels. Immune abnormalities, including allergy, are also commonly observed in this disorder. Allergy may play a role in pathogenesis of Autism wherein immune responses to allergens may induce the production of brain auto-antibodies found in many autistic children. Hyper-serotonemia may be the reason behind the increased frequency of allergic manifestations in autistic children through reduction of T-helper 1-type cytokines. The study investigated the possible connection between hyper-serotonemia and the increased frequency of allergic manifestations in 40 autistic and 40 healthy matched children. Autistic children had significantly higher serum serotonin levels than controls [125 (250.75) vs. 41.5 (41.5) ng/mL, P < 0.001]. Fifty five percent (22/40) of autistic children had elevated serum serotonin. Allergic manifestations (bronchial asthma, atopic dermatitis and allergic rhinitis) were elicited in 45% of autistic patients which were significantly higher than controls (10%, P < 0.001). Moreover, autistic patients with allergic manifestations had significantly higher serum serotonin levels than those without (P < 0.001). Furthermore, there was a significant positive correlation between serum serotonin and total immunoglobulin E levels in autistic patients (r = 0.8, P < 0.001). In conclusion, hyper-serotonemia may be a contributing factor to the increased frequency of allergic manifestations in some autistic children. Inclusion of serum serotonin levels as a correlate may be useful in future immune studies in Autism to help unravel the long-standing mystery of hyper-serotonemia and its possible role in the pathophysiology of this disorder. In addition, the effect of blood serotonin lowering drugs in hyper-serotonemic autistic children, on amelioration of allergic manifestations and immune abnormalities, should be studied [25].

In summary, there are many comorbid factors that may play a roll in the cause of allergy induced Autism. It is likely that the breadth and scope of such comorbid interactions affect the degree of atypicality within Autism Spectrum Disorders.

REFERENCES

[1]   Michael Waldman, Sean Nicholson, Nodir Adilov. Does Television Cause Autism?
      http://www.johnson.cornell.edu/faculty/profiles/Waldman/AUTISM-WALDMAN-NICHOLSON-ADILOV.pdf

[2]   Nila J. Rosen, Cathleen K. Yoshida, Lisa A. Croen. (2007). Infection in the First 2 Years of Life and Autism Spectrum Disorders. *Pediatrics. Volume 119*, Number 1, pages e61-e69.

[3]   Stephen M. Edelson: Allergies and Food Sensitivities; Center for the Study of Autism, Salem, Oregon. Autism Today, http://www.autismtoday.com/allergiesfood.htm

[4]   Doctor's Guide. (1997). Global Edition: Mild Infections Linked to Allergy and Asthma, http://www.pslgroup.com/dg/1ECDE.htm

[5]   T.W. McDade, C.W. Kuzawa, L.S. Adair, *et al.* (2004). Prenatal and early postnatal environments are significant predictors of total immunoglobulin E

concentrations in Filipino adolescents. *Clinical and Experimental Allergy. Volume 34*, pages 44-50.

[6] Vitali Pool, M. Miles Braun, John M. Kelso, et al. (2002). Prevalence of Anti-Gelatin IgE Antibodies in People with Anaphylaxis After Measles-Mumps-Rubella in the United States. *Pediatrics. Volume 1-110*, Number 6, page e71.

[7] Denis Peronnet, Anesthesiology Department, Center hospitalier - Boulevard de 1 Hopital - 71018 Macon France: The role of Oxytocin in natural-latex Allergy during Cesarean-Section. http://www.csen.com/ anesthesia/ latex.htm.

[8] Kai-Chien Chang, David A. Hammer. (1999). The Forward Rate of Binding of Surface-Tethered Reactants; Effects of Relative Motion between Two Surfaces. *Journal of Biophysics. Volume 76*, Number 3. pages 1280-1292

[9] Bjorksten B, Sepp E, Julge K, Voort Mikelsaar M. (2001). Allergy development and the intestinal microflora during the first year of like; *Journal of Allergy and Clinical Immunology, Volume 108*, Number 4, pages 516-520.

[10] Nicholas M. F. Oyane. (2005). Sleep disturbances in adolescents and young adults with Autism and Aspergers syndrome. *Autism. Volume 9*, Number 1, pages 83-94.

[11] John J, We M-F, Boehmer L, Siegel JM. (2004). "Cataplexy-Active Neurons in the Hypothalamus: Implications for the Role of Histamine in Sleep and Waking Behavior." *Neuron. Volume 42*, pages 619-634.

[12] Osamu Hayaishi. (2000). Molecular mechanisms of sleep-wake regulation: roles of prostaglandins D2 and E2, *B Biol. Sci. Volume 355*. Number 1394, pages 275-280.

[13] Evangelisto M. (1997). Latex allergy: the downside of standard precautions. *Today's Surg Nurse. Volume 19*, pages 28–33.

[14] Liu CA, Wang CL, Chuang H, Ou CY, *et al.* ( ). Prenatal prediction of infant atopy by maternal but not paternal total IgE levels. *Journal of Allergy and Clinical Immunology. NV, Volume 112*, Number 5, pages 899-904.

[15] Stephen M. Canfield, *et al.* (2008). Total and specific IgE associations between New York City Head Start children and their parents, *The Journal of Allergy and Clinical Immunology. Volume 12*, Issue 6, pages 1422-1427.e4.

[16] Neiderberger V, Niggemann B, Kraft D, et al. (2002). Evolution of IgM, IgE, IgG (1-4) antibody responses in early childhood monitored with

recombinant allergen components. *European Journal of Immunology. Volume 32*, Number 2, pages 576-84.

[17] IgE levels modulate expression of IgE receptors on dendritic cells (2003). *Journal of Allergy and Clinical Immunology. Volume 112*, pages 1147-1154.

[18] Alexander C. Drew *et.al.* (2004). Hypoallergenic Variants of the Major Latex Allergens Hev b-6.01Retaining Human T Lymphocyte Reactivity. *The Journal of Immunology. Volume 173*, pages 5872-5879.

[19] William Walsh, Metallothionein Dysfunction, Pfeiffer Treatment Center. http://www.springboard4health.com/notebook/health_autism2.html#2

[20] Kaede Gomi, Fu-Gang Zhu, and Jean S. Marshall. (2000). Prostaglandin E2 Selectively Enhances the IgE-Mediated Production of IL-6 and Granulocyte_Macrophage Colony-Stimulating Factor by Mast Cells Through an EP1/EP2-Dependent Mechanism. *The Journal of Immunology. Volume 165*, pages 6545-6552.

[21] Naomi Eguchi, Toshiaki Minami, Naoki Shirafuji, et al. (1999). Lack of tactile pain (allodynia) in lipocalin-type prostaglandin D synthase-deficient mice. *Proc National Academy of Science United States of America. Volume 96*, Number 2, pages 726–730.

[22] Morley, J. E., Kay, N. E., Solomon, G. F., et al. (1987). Neuropeptides: conductors of the immune orchestra, *Life Science. Volume 41*, Number 5, pages 527-44.

[23] Shaaban A. Mousa, Bapaiah P. Cheppudira, Mohammed Shaqura, et al. (2007). Nerve growth factor governs the enhanced ability of opioids to suppress inflammatory pain. Volume 130, Number 2, pages 502-513.

[24] Croonenberghs et al. (2000). Peripheral Markers of Serotonergic and Noradrenergic Function in Post-Pubertal, Caucasian Males with Autistic Disorder. *Neuropsychopharmacology. Volume 22*, pages 275-283.

[25] Gehan A. Mostafa, Dalia F. EL-Sherif, Rasha T. Hamza, Abeer AL Shehab. (2008). Hyperserotonemia in Egyptian autistic children: Relation to allergic manifestations. *Journal of Pediatric Neurology. Volume 6*, Number 3, pages 227-236.

Chapter IX

GOVERNMENT

The infant is at the center of the world... -Edward J. Bardon MD

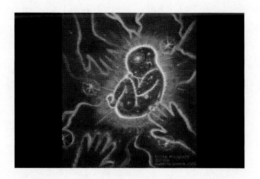

During adolescence, Dain's relationship with his mother and younger brother was often strained and occasionally violent. Although his mother always treated him with the greatest care and respect; it can only be speculated that the frustration of isolation accompanied with sensory over-load caused him intense irritability. On one occasion while agitated and next to his mother, he sank his teeth into her face. For her, seconds seemed to turn into minutes as the intense grip failed to release. The swollen indentation on her cheek faded away after several hours but the physical attack caused a mental scar. Unconditional love, sympathy, and compassion eventually replaced shock and anger with understanding; although she would always be on guard in the future. In another family incident, Dain's younger brother learned to stay several arm lengths away because without provocation or warning, Dain would suddenly hit his brother on the head causing painful tears and fear.

DOES OUR DEPENDENCE ON NATURAL-LATEX AFFECT THE REGULATION OF HEVEA BRASILIENSIS?

Government agencies including the Environmental Protection Agency and the Food & Drug Administration are aware of some of the hazards associated with natural-latex.

Will future government mandates set guidelines on allergenic protein content in natural-latex?

Although many of the issues associated with natural-latex are well documented and understood, industrial societies magnificent exploitation and comfortable dependence on such a material continues to stress human health. Government agencies who have been emboldened to guide infant health and safety have shown contradictions in policy with regard to natural-latex.

Environmental Protection Agency

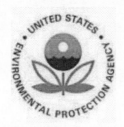

In 2008, a citizen petition was filed under section 21 of the Toxic Substances Control Act requesting that the Director issue a regulation that prohibits the use and distribution in commerce of Hevea brasiliensis natural-latex adhesives having total protein content greater than 200 micrograms per dry weight of latex. The petitions intent was that implementation of an Environmental Protection Agency regulation that guides adhesive manufacturer's to use a Hevea brasiliensis natural-latex adhesive that satisfies such requirements may affect the incidence of natural-latex allergy during pregnancy and allergy induced Autism in neonates [1].

The term "toxic substance" is often defined by the designation LD50 which is a measure of how much constitutes a lethal dose. For example, in animal testing the dose administered that kills half the test population is referred to as the LD50. Many of the proteins in Hevea brasiliensis natural-latex are considered chronic non-infectious agents (i.e., allergens). Their hazards are related too the intensity and duration of an immune response based on exposure and genetic influences. Therefore, LD50 data on allergenic proteins are extremely difficult to quantify even though individuals have died from anaphylactic shock after exposure.

Congress included a citizens' petition provision in the Toxic Substance Control Act specifically so that the Environmental Protection Agency might be prodded into action:

The responsiveness of government is a critical concern and the citizens' petition provision will help to protect against lax enforcement [2].

The provision was modeled on the Consumer Product Safety Act, passed in 1972 [3]. Ironically, five years later, Congress repealed the citizens' petition provision in the Consumer Product Safety Act [4].

Under section 21, any person may petition the Administrator to initiate a proceeding for the issuance, amendment, or repeal of a rule under section 4, 6, or 8 or an order under section 5(e) or 6(b)(2). A petition filed under section 21 must be filed with the Environmental Protection Agency Headquarters and must include the facts supporting the Environmental Protection Agency action under one of the applicable sections of the Toxic Substance Control Act [5]. The Environmental Protection Agency must either grant or deny the petition within 90 days of the filing of the petition [6]. If the Environmental Protection Agency grants the petition, the Environmental Protection Agency must promptly commence a proceeding under the appropriate section of the Toxic Substance Control Act [7]. If the Environmental Protection Agency instead denies the petition, the Environmental Protection Agency must publish its reasons for denying the petition in the Federal Register [8].

A petitioner may file an action in a district court if the Environmental Protection Agency either denies a petition or the Environmental Protection Agency fails to either grant or deny a petition within 90 days of the filing of the petition [9]. A court must order the Environmental Protection Agency to initiate the action requested by the petitioner if the petitioner demonstrates by a preponderance of the evidence the following elements. For a petition for a rule under section 4 or an order under section 5, the petitioner must show that: (I) information available to the Environmental Protection Agency "is insufficient to permit a reasoned evaluation of the health and environmental effects of the chemical substance" in question, and (II) without such information the substance "may present an unreasonable risk to health or the environment" or the substance is or will be produced in substantial quantities and enters or may be anticipated to enter the environment in substantial quantities or there is or may be significant or substantial human exposure to the substance [10].

For a petition brought to compel the issuance of a rule under section 6 or 8, or an order under section 6(b)(2), a petitioner must prove that there is a reasonable basis for concluding that a rule or order is necessary to protect health or the environment against an unreasonable risk of injury to health or the environment [11]. A court may allow the Environmental Protection Agency to defer issuance of a rule or order sought by a petitioner if a court makes two findings: the extent of the risk to health or the environment alleged by the petitioner is less than the extent of the risks which the Environmental Protection Agency is addressing under TSCA, and the Environmental Protection Agency has insufficient resources to take the action sought by the petitioner [12]. A court may award costs and attorneys fees if it determines that such an award is appropriate [13].

The citizen petition was denied on June 3rd, 2008 for the following reasons:

Natural-latex adhesives comprise a very small portion of the adhesive industry. They are grouped by the United States Census under the "natural base glues and adhesives" product category, which comprises the smallest (less than three percent) of the United States adhesive manufacturing industry;

The petition does not present facts establishing that latex adhesives containing any specific level of protein present an unreasonable risk;

According to the American Society for Testing and Materials, "although this method detects antigenic proteins, it should not be considered as a measure of allergenic proteins because correlation of protein/antigen levels with the level of allergenic proteins has not been fully established;

The petitioner only speculates that implementation of an Environmental Protection Agency regulation may affect the incidence and prevalence of latex allergy and allergy induced Autism in neonates;

A United States Consumer Product Safety Commission determination suggests that the risks associated with natural-latex, principally Hevea brasiliensis natural-latex, are relatively insubstantial, and does not support a conclusion that any risk is unreasonable;

The petition does not discuss any special risks posed by natural-latex adhesives (in comparison to other natural rubber latex products or other adhesives), does not describe the contexts in which one might be exposed to natural-latex adhesives or why those exposures are of concern to the general population, and does not provide any other information why adhesives are of particularly concern;

The petition contains little information on the relative importance of Hevea brasiliensis natural-latex adhesives as a source of infant exposure;

The petitioner has not provided evidence showing that prohibiting Hevea brasiliensis natural-latex adhesives that did not meet this standard would be the least burdensome requirement;

A regulation requiring reduced protein content in Hevea brasiliensis natural-latex adhesives is unlikely to significantly contribute to reducing Hevea brasiliensis natural-latex allergy in the general population; and

Natural-latex free synthetic alternatives are available, but these alternatives are more expensive and may not perform as well as Hevea brasiliensis natural-latex adhesives. As evidence that substitutes may create their own risk, many synthetic elastomers contain traces of carcinogens, and the production of vinyl gloves, a major substitute for latex gloves, increases the risk of dioxin releases into the atmosphere [14].

In response, the petitioner respectfully disagreed with the Assistant Administrator and presented the following rebuttal:

In the petition it states, "Continued efforts in the United States have been undertaken to identify sources of Hevea brasiliensis natural-latex in order to minimize release into the environment. For example, in the medical industry, efforts continue to substantially eliminate natural-latex in the health care environment. Specifically, Johns Hopkins Hospital recently announced in 2008 that it will no longer use nearly all medical natural-latex products. Medical products that contain Hevea brasiliensis natural-latex adhesives are targeted for exclusion. In the petition denial, the Assistant Administrator fails to recognize or address the significant exclusionary practice described above.

In continuation, it was disclosed in the petition that consumer groups are calling for warning labels on food packaging containing latex (i.e., natural latex adhesives), saying the substance poses a potential threat to people with allergic sensitivities. A well published article entitled,

Deadly Latex Evading Lax Food Labeling Laws presents a British study which shows that food-contamination from latex may be a dangerous health risk for both children and adults. In the petition denial, the Assistant Administrator fails to recognize or address the health risk that natural latex adhesives pose when used in food packaging.

Innovative and forward thinking companies like Vystar Corporation have demonstrated that allergenic proteins can be substantially removed (e.g., less than 10 $\mu g/dm^2$) from Hevea brasiliensis natural-latex to provide adhesives having enhanced non-allergenicity while retaining effective bonding characteristics - The petitioner submits that it would not be an undue burden for the Assistant Administrator to re-evaluate the validity of the Citizen Petition in light of the Vystar Corporation protein-extraction technology described above.

The non-differentiation of antigenic protein (innate and/or adaptive immune response) versus an allergenic protein (adaptive immune response), according to the American Society for Testing and Materials, is moot in that both protein classifications elicit an adverse immune response.

The petitioner agrees with a public comment by a manufacturer of natural-latex and natural-latex-free bandages that stated, "because it would go a long way in preventing allergic reactions that have become more common....".

The Rubber Manufacturers Association noted that in the long history of Hevea brasiliensis natural-latex harvest and use, and in the course of multiple government inquiries into latex allergy, no one had observed a link between Hevea brasiliensis natural-latex and Autism. The petitioner agreed and stated, "When we let down a child that has atopy we're all to blame." Furthermore, the Rubber Manufacturers Association responded to the petition as follows: "Latex rubber may even *reduce* the symptoms of Autism, according to one member of the Autistic Society who has successfully used 'trance suits' i.e., inflatable natural latex rubber suits".

In a recent study entitled, *Allergic manifestations in autistic children: Relations to disease severity*, research showed that allergy may play a role in the pathogenesis of Autism wherein allergic immune responses to some proteins (e.g., dietary protein and natural latex) may induce the production of brain auto-antibodies, which are found in many autistic children [15].

In 2004, the U.S. Consumer Product Safety Commission denied petition HP00-2 requesting a rule declaring natural rubber latex to be a strong sensitizer. The Honorable Thomas H. Moore (Commissioner) stated, "Nevertheless, it would behoove manufacturers of natural rubber latex to take steps to reduce the level of proteins that consumers can come into contact with, whether or not the end product is a medical device" [16].

As part of its focus on children's exposure to the antigenic/allergenic proteins in Hevea brasiliensis, the petitioner would welcome the opportunity to discuss potential partnership approaches to data collection and product stewardship.

The Environmental Protection Agency responded to the rebuttal in a letter dated July 18th, 2008, the Office of Pollution Prevention and Toxics director stated:

"The Environmental Protection Agency was aware that it is possible to produce low-allergen natural rubber latex";

"Please be assured that the Environmental Protection Agency carefully considered this information, as well as much other information, during its review of your petition"; and

"The Environmental Protection Agency does not have any current plans to collect data or conduct a product stewardship program on natural rubber latex adhesives".

In the public interest, the petitioner sent a request to the Minnesota Attorney General to file a lawsuit, on behalf of the State of Minnesota, in an effort to reverse the Environmental Protection Agency denial of the petition. The Attorney General's office responded in a letter dated August 5th, 2008, "Because the Attorney General's Office is not authorized to represent private citizens, I cannot file a lawsuit on your behalf". The petitioner wrote the following rebuttal:

It is well known that the Environmental Protection Agency is proactively participating in the recycling of Hevea brasiliensis natural-latex, without regard for the antigenic protein content therein. The ambiguous phrase "unreasonable risk", used to deny the citizen petition, appears to be burdened with a conflict of interest. Specifically, the Environmental Protection Agency promotes the use of ground rubber tires in recreational applications and states, "The material can absorb much of the impact from falls providing added safety for children". The Environmental Protection Agency should be exploring ways to reduce child exposure to the antigenic proteins (i.e., *Hev-b* proteins) that are inherent in ground rubber tires and natural rubber latex adhesives. The petitioner respectfully requested that the Environmental Protection Agency reconsider their participation in the continuous proliferation of Hevea brasiliensis natural rubber latex.

In the prevention of allergy induced Autism and mental health disorders during child development, we should question if such agencies should be in the business of the proliferation of natural-latex, without regard for the allergenic proteins therein.

Furthermore, the petitioner submitted an editorial to the Centers for Disease Control entitled, *Antigenic Proteins and Government Policy* (Preventing Chronic Disease - Manuscript PCD-08-0168) in an effort to communicate issues with Government policy related to the antigenic proteins inherent in Hevea brasiliensis natural-latex. The editorial is a review on how Government agencies, who have been emboldened to guide health & safety, have shown contradictions in policy with Hevea brasiliensis natural-latex.

On August 27, 2008 the article was rejected by the acting Editor-in-Chief and it was stated,

"It has been evaluated by the editors, and unfortunately the topic is outside the scope of this journal"

The United States Environmental Protection Agency is also involved in the promotion of recycled natural-latex [17]. The use of crumb rubber from recycled tires has been touted by the Environmental Protection Agency and a number of state environmental agencies as having beneficial impact on the environment. A specific example wherein the United States Government is involved in the recycling of natural-latex, without regard for the antigenic proteins, is in U.S. Pat. 6,407,144. In the *Government Interests* section of the patent it states, "The United States Government has rights to this invention pursuant to contract number DE-AC09-96-SR18500 between the U.S. Department of Energy and Westinghouse Savannah". The shift toward radial tires, which use a higher percentage of natural-latex than bias-ply tires, has resulted in an increase in natural-latex consumption over the past twenty years. We should question if the recycling of natural-latex, without regard for the antigenic proteins therein, is good government policy when considering the health and safety of all Americans.

A study indicates that allergies are increasing. A new test that identifies allergen-specific IgE antibodies in blood samples gives quantifiable evidence that allergies are increasing in both frequency and severity, according to findings presented at the 61st annual meeting of the American Academy of Allergy,

Asthma, and Immunology [18]. One may reasonably suggest that exposure to the allergens in natural-latex has been a major contributor. In industrial societies, such allergenic proteins may indeed be the most pervasive allergens of the late twentieth century.

Food and Drug Administration

Currently, infant products formed from Hevea brasiliensis natural-latex are not required by law to disclose protein content. For example, manufacturers of baby bottle nipples and pacifiers do not display antigenic protein warnings or protein content information on their packaging. Health and safety is often compromised in that rubber manufacturers are not required to disclose such information.

The Food and Drug Administration is aware of some of the hazards associated with Hevea brasiliensis natural-latex, based on medical latex glove issues. In January, 1998, Public Citizen and Dr. Timothy Sullivan, Professor of Medicine at Emory and Head of the subsection of Allergy and Immunology at the Emory Clinic, petitioned the Food and Drug Administration to ban powdered latex gloves because of their significant dangers and because of the fact that safer alternatives are available. At that time, the Food and Drug Administration had already been studying this issue for at least two years. When the Food and Drug Administration published the July 30, 1999 Federal Register notice announcing the reclassification of powdered latex gloves, the agency also rejected the petition to ban powdered latex gloves [19].

The Food and Drug Administration has provided guidance on the hazards of medical gloves and medical devices formed from Hevea brasiliensis natural-latex. For example, the Food and Drug Administration requires medical glove manufacturers to identify on the package labeling that natural-latex is used. Furthermore, the Food and Drug Administration requires that all medical devices containing natural-latex to be labeled as such and to carry a caution that natural-latex can cause allergic reactions.

In 2007, a citizen petition requested that the Commissioner issue a regulation for Hevea brasiliensis natural-latex, used in the manufacture of infant products, wherein said latex meets the minimum standards of protein content based on The American Society for Testing and Materials D1076-06 (Category 4) that defines latex containing less than 200 micrograms total protein per gram of dry weight of natural-latex.

In a letter from the Food and Drug Administration dated July, 18, 2008, the Director - Office of Food Additive Safety - wrote,

"The purpose of this letter is to advise you, in accordance with 21 CFR 10.30(e), that we have not reached a decision within 180 days of the filing of the petition because of the limited availability of resources and other agency priorities."

Natural-latex allergy continues to be a serious health issue. In 2008, the Food and Drug Administration failed to make a decision on the health and safety of infant products formed from Hevea brasiliensis natural-latex.

On April 23, 2008, the Food and Drug Administration (FDA) cleared for marketing the Yulex Patient examination gloves, the first medical device made from guayule latex which is non-Hevea brasiliensis natural-latex having reduced allergenic protein content.

United States Patent and Trademarks

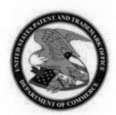

In 2007, a United States Patent was filed entitled, *Method of Natural Rubber Latex Avoidance to affect the development of Autism Spectrum Disorders* [20].

The patent intent is that implementation of a method that guides consumers to avoid exposure to Hevea brasiliensis natural-latex will affect the incidence of latex allergy during pregnancy and affect the atypicality of allergy induced Autism.

The invention discloses a method that can be used to substantially reduce immunoglobulin-E mediated reaction antibodies induced by natural-latex, which may affect the development of Autism Spectrum Disorders. The method comprising the steps of:

Providing at least one individual at conception;
Providing an environment for said individual wherein the environment is substantially free of materials formed from natural-latex; then
Allowing said individual to develop in said environment for at least about ten years.

It is written that surprisingly, the method can be used to substantially reduce hyper adaptive immunity and cross-reactivity from natural-latex. Furthermore, it is surmised that the inventive method can be used to substantially reduce immunoglobulin-E mediated reaction antibodies that have been induced by the allergens present in Hevea brasiliensis natural-latex. It is further surmised that adult females having a positive immunoglobulin-E response to the allergens in Hevea brasiliensis natural-latex during pregnancy are more likely to have offspring that experience developmental, learning and behavioral disabilities including Autism Spectrum Disorders. It is still further surmised that a developing fetus has an increased predisposition to an adverse immune response if one or both parents are adversely affected by the allergens in Hevea brasiliensis natural-latex. It is finally surmised that an immature nervous system having a positive immunoglobulin-E immune response to the allergens in Hevea brasiliensis natural-latex are more susceptible to food allergens and non-food allergens. The frequency and intensity of the immunoglobulin-E mediated reaction antibodies induced by such dissimilar allergens that cross-react can adversely affect the severity of the Autism Spectrum Disorder.

The patent application was rejected by the Patent Examiner and an *Appeal Brief* was filed to the *Patent Board of Appeals* summarizing the reasons for a reversal of the rejection and subsequent allowance of the claims. Highlights from the *Appeal Brief* are as follows:

In rejection of the patent claims, the Examiner stated,

"The current point of view in the art is such that causes of Autism Spectrum Disorders (Autism, Aspergers, and Rett syndrome) are currently unknown; however, Autism remains among the most heritable developmental disorders."

The applicants' disagreed and stated,
There is no scientific evidence of record establishing that Autism remains among the most heritable developmental disorders."

The Examiner further states,

> "The information presented in the patent is limited at best to the disclosure of a working hypothesis that elimination of natural-latex from the environment of an individual would affect (in a positive way) the development of Autism. There appears to be no further support disclosed at the time of filing, in the form of references to prior art on the cause of Autism, or any experimental data, which would link Hevea brasiliensis natural-latex, immunoglobulin-E antibodies and Autism Spectrum Disorders, or any other scientific reasoning that would provide for a skilled practitioner as how to practice the patent."

The Applicants' disagreed and stated,

> "There is no prior art references that link Hevea brasiliensis natural-latex exposure and Autism Spectrum Disorder. An area of research on the cause of Autism Spectrum Disorders, currently in its infancy, is allergy induced Autism. The patent provides an advantage which never before was appreciated as it relates to allergy induced Autism in that it discloses a method that can effectively reduce cross-react immune responses (e.g., food allergies) induced by Hevea brasiliensis natural-latex exposure, that can trigger immune hyperactivity affecting the incidence of allergy induced Autism. The Applicants use scientific reasoning to teach that the method can be used to substantially reduce immunoglobulin-E mediated reaction antibodies induced by Hevea brasiliensis natural-latex. The Applicants use scientific reasoning to teach that elevated immunoglobulin-E antibodies (positive immunoglobulin-E response) usually indicates an allergy and that exposure to Hevea brasiliensis natural-latex should be avoided during neurological development. Finally, the Applicants argue that scientific reasoning is used to teach that the frequency and intensity of such exposure to Hevea brasiliensis natural-latex may increase the likelihood of an Immunoglobulin-E antibody response affecting neurological development through allergy induced Autism."

The Examiner further rejected the patent based on the absence of working examples and stated,

> "Working examples could include practicing the method using an art-accepted model for Autism, such as an animal model or *in vitro*

experiments, which would support the method design and be predictive of the claimed invention."

The Applicants' disagreed and stated,

"Animal models have not shown utility in that Autism is recognized exclusively as a human disorder based on the American Psychiatric Association's *Diagnostic and Statistical Manual of Mental Disorders IV*. The Applicants argue that *in Vitro* experiments have not shown utility in that effective and reliable laboratory simulation of brain neurological development and functioning remains elusive with current technologies. Applicants argue that there is no effective or reliable art-accepted model that is predictive for Autism Spectrum Disorders. Finally, the Applicants argue that the exclusionary method uses scientific reasoning and that anecdotal evidence provides enablement, guidance, and effectively teaches the method of the patent allowing those skilled in the art to practice it."

The Examiner further rejected the patent and stated,

"The patent must teach those skilled in the art how to make and use the full scope of the invention without undue experimentation and there must be sufficient disclosure, either through illustrative examples or terminology, to teach those of ordinary skill how to make and how to use the invention as broadly as it is claimed."

The Applicants' disagreed and stated,

"The specification teaches what type of natural-latex (i.e., Hevea brasiliensis) should be avoided. The Applicants teach at what biological age Hevea brasiliensis natural-latex should be avoided such as from conception to twenty-one years of age. The Applicants teach the type of products that may contain Hevea brasiliensis natural-latex including baby bottle nipples. The Applicants teach what environments Hevea brasiliensis natural-latex may be present including day care facilities and schools. Finally, the Applicants argue that the skilled artisan is given sufficient guidance on how to practice the method of the patent without undue experimentation."

The Examiners further rejected the patent claims and stated,

"Reciting the term "to affect" which is a relative term renders the patent indefinite. The term "to affect" encompasses both negative and positive effect, and the patent fails to define which affect is intended."

The Applicants disagreed and stated,

"Autism is considered a spectrum disorder; it would be medically unethical (i.e., non-therapeutic) to provide a patent that increases its incidence. Therefore, those skilled in the art would recognize that the term *affect* indicates a positive effect."

In summary, the patent is now under appeal and the *Patent Board of Appeals* must determine if scientific reasoning can be used to validate a method of natural-latex exclusion, affecting the incidence and atypicality of allergy induce Autism.

REFERENCES

[1]   Citizen Petition EPA-HQ-OPPT-2008-0273; FRL-8368-4, March 6, 2008, http://www.epa.gov/EPA-TOX/2008/April/Day-25/t9041.htm

[2]   S. Rep. No. 94-698 at 13 (1976), reprinted in H. Comm. on Interstate and Foreign Commerce, Legislative History of the Toxic Substances Control Act at 169 (1976).

[3]   *Id.* at 12, Legis. Hist. at 168, referring to Pub. L. 92-753 (1972), § 10, 86 Stat. 1217.

[4]   Consumer Product Safety Amendments of 1981, § 1210, Title XII, Subtitle A of the Omnibus Budget Reconciliation Act of 1981, Pub. L. 97-35 (1981), 95 Stat. 721.

[5]   TSCA § 21(b)(1), 15 U.S.C. § 2620(b)(1).

[6]   TSCA § 21(b)(3), 15 U.S.C. § 2620(b)(3).

[7]   TSCA § 21(b)(3), 15 U.S.C. § 2620(b)(3).

[8]   TSCA § 21(b)(3), 15 U.S.C. § 2620(b)(3).

[9]   TSCA § 21(b)(4)(A), 15 U.S.C. § 2620(b)(4)(A). Such an action must be filed within 60 days of EPA's denial of the petition, or within 60 days after the expiration of the 90 day period in which EPA failed to either grant or deny the petition.

[10] TSCA § 21(b)(4)(B)(i), 15 U.S.C. § 2620(b)(4)(B)(i).

[11] TSCA § 21(b)(4)(B)(ii), 15 U.S.C. § 2620(b)(4)(B)(ii).

[12] TSCA § 21(b)(4)(B), 15 U.S.C. § 2620(b)(4)(B).

[13] TSCA § 21(b)(4)(C), 15 U.S.C. § 2620(b)(4)(C).

[14] Natural Rubber Latex Adhesives; Disposition of EPA-HQ-OPPT-2008-0273; FRL-8368-4, June 9, 2008 (Volume 73, Number 111), http://edocket.access.gpo.gov/2008/E8-12850.htm

[15] Gehan A. Mostafa, Rasha T. Hamza, Heba H. El-shahawi. (2008). Allergic manifestations in autistic children: Relation to disease Severity. *Journal of Pediatric Neurology. Volume 6*, Number 2, pages 115-123.

[16] Statement of the Honorable Thomas H. Moore on Petition HP 00-2; Requesting a Rule Declaring Natural Rubber Latex to be a Strong Sensitizer. April 30, 2004. http://www.cpsc.gov/library/foia/f oia04/ petition/ rubberla.pdf

[17] Environmental Protection Agency website, Science/Technology, Management of Scrap Tires. http://www.epa.gov/osw/conserve/ materials/ tires/science.htm

[18] Paula Moyer. (2005). AAAAI: Allergen-Specific IgE Test Confirms Increase in Allergy Frequency and Severity. http://www.pslgroup.com/ dg/24b7ce.htm

[19] Sidney M. Wolfe, Director, Public Citizen's Health Research Group, Concerning FDA's Proposed Regulation on Powdered Latex Gloves, Docket No. 98N-0313. http://www.citizen.org/publications/release. cfm?ID=6707

[20] U.S. Patent & Trademark Office, Patent Application 20070034214A1, February 15, 2007, http://appft1.uspto.gov/netacgi/nph-Parser?Sect1= PTO2& Sect2=HITOFF&p=1&u=%2Fnetahtml%2FPTO%2Fsearch-bool.html&r=1&f=G&l=50&co1=AND&d=PG01&s1=dochniak&OS=dochnia k&RS=dochniak

Chapter X

SCIENCE

A new scientific truth does not triumph by convincing its opponents and making them see the light, but rather because its opponents eventually die, and a new generation grows up that is familiar with it. -Thomas Samuel Kuhn

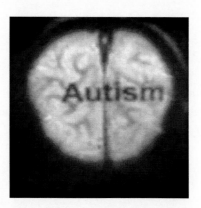

From kindergarten through high school, many professionals have participated in Dain's Regressive Autism journey and have used great determination, skill, and passion to try to bring learning into his life. In the first few years, facilitated learning was the only way to get Dain's attention. The teacher assisted Dain by holding his hand(s) and directing their movement to accomplish a task. As an example, it took several years to teach Dain how to pick up crayons and place them in a plastic container. The teachers' facilitated and rewarded his progress; patiently awaiting the day he would consistently initiate and complete the task independently. Sometimes, their brief success came when Dain performed the task only to never do it again. Herculean efforts by these many professionals have failed to accomplish targeted learning goals; his cognitive abilities remain essentially untestable.

HAS NATURAL-LATEX SENSITIVITY CAUSED AN INCREASED INCIDENCE OF ALLERGY INDUCED AUTISM?

In 1964 the World Medical Association developed a code of research ethics that came to be known as the Declaration of Helsinki. It was a reinterpretation of the Nuremberg Code, with an eye to medical research with therapeutic intent. Thus, human experimental research directed at prenatal/neonatal/infant induced immune responses to the allergens in natural-latex is unethical and prohibited based on non-therapeutic intent.

Can Animal Studies be used to Falsify the Allergy Induced Autism hypothesis?

The pursuit of animal studies lacks justification in that Autism Spectrum Disorders are exclusively a human disorder based on the American Psychiatric Association's *Diagnostic and Statistical Manual of Mental Disorders IV*.

Can *In-vitro* Experiments Falsify the Allergy Induced Autism Hypothesis?

Genetic studies may show utility in deciphering clues to the immune system, but, the current unpredictability of *Hev-b* allergenic-protein insult, immunoglobulin-E cross reactivity, and other comorbid factors including viral induced hyper-immunity associated with non-infectious antigenic protein insult adds complexity to the cause of allergy induced Autism.

Can *Hev-b* Allergenic-Protein Exclusionary Practice be used to Falsify the Allergy Induced Autism Hypothesis?

Yes, limit *Hev-b* allergenic-protein exposure during neurological development and monitor the global incidence and/or the degree of atypicality of Autism Spectrum Disorders thereafter.

The term "science" is often described as the search for truth. In mathematics, we have been taught that the purity of numbers gives us an objective tool in the search for scientific truth. Adaptive immunity is static and therefore reported incidence of natural-latex allergies in the general population may be misunderstood. In industrialized societies, it may be understood that the antigenic proteins in natural-latex have caused an immune response in most individual's at some point in their life based on its prevalence and repeated exposure.

Allergy induced Autism based on natural-latex allergy is an etiology that must be dealt with carefully in that inappropriate allergy testing could be harmful. For example, direct exposure allergy-tests (e.g., the skin prick test, patch test, challenge test) when used on neonates is a conundrum in that insult to the *Hev-b* proteins, to determine if an allergy exists, may induce sensitivity to atopic individuals - the threshold of sensitivity to such protein(s) is unknown even though some of these tests use minute quantities.

In other allergy research, allergy immunotherapy has been shown to be somewhat effective wherein a predetermined injection/dosage schedule of the allergenic protein is used to gradually shift the immune response from adaptive immunity (immunoglobulin-E) to innate immunity (immunoglobulin-G). Unfortunately, the un-predictability of cross reactions with homologous proteins makes this procedure risky for atopic children.

It would be beneficial to have a *Hev-b* protein vaccine which effectively triggers an immunoglobulin-G response instead of an immunoglobulin-E response, especially during neonatal/infant development. In speculation, it may be useful to alter the tertiary structure of the allergenic protein while maintaining its primary and secondary structure. For example, most naturally occurring proteins are formed from L-amino acids which provide a specific stereochemistry essential for epitope/receptor binding. Engineering the synthesis of *Hev-b* allergenic-proteins inclusive with D-amino acids may inhibit the *Hev-b* allergenic-protein/immunoglobulin-E binding characteristic possibly shifting the immune response to immunoglobulin-G. Thus, steriochemical modification of allergenic proteins may be a useful method to inhibit the adaptive immune response.

Alternatively, it is unknown how the density of an allergenic protein affects the adaptive immune response. In further speculation, it may be useful to alter the density of the allergenic protein while maintaining its primary, secondary, and tertiary structure by replacing an effective number of hydrogen atoms on the allergenic protein with deuterium atoms. Since deuterium is heavier that hydrogen the density of the allergenic protein may be altered enough to cause an innate immune response instead of an adaptive immune response. Thus, allergenic proteins that have been deuterated may be useful in allergy immunotherapy.

Can the Timing, Frequency, Intensity, and Type of Exposure to Allergenic Proteins Affect the Incidence of Autism Spectrum Disorders?

It is the opinion of the authors that adaptive immunity is an important part of Mankind's neuro-cognitive evolution. In a developing nervous system, allergies can cause atypical neural growth and atypical synaptic pruning. The authors have spent much effort exploring allergy induced Autism using biological models and theoretical models of the adaptive immune system. From an evolutionary standpoint, hyper-adaptive immunity appears to be an important immunological feature that differentiates mankind from all other creatures. It is this immunity that allows the brain to reach extremes in cognition from exceptional brilliance to the mentally impaired. Natural-latex has subjected atopic individuals to an extreme mixture of allergenic proteins resulting in atypical adaptive-immunity and atypical neurological development. The medical profession (i.e., iatrogenic allergies) has over-exposed atopic prenates/neonates/infants to the allergenic proteins in natural-latex causing an increased incidence of allergy induced Autism.

In 2009, a study of California data found that the reported incidence of Autism rose 7- to 8-fold from the early 1990s to 2007, and that changes in diagnostic criteria, inclusion of milder cases, and earlier age of diagnosis probably explain only a 4.25-fold increase [1]. Another 2009 California study found that the reported increases are unlikely to be explained by changes in how qualifying condition codes for Autism were recorded [2].

REFERENCES

[1]   Hertz-Picciotto I, Delwiche L (2009). The rise in Autism and the role of age at diagnosis. *Epidemiology, Volume 20*, number 1, pages 84–90.

[2]   Grether JK, Rosen NJ, Smith KS, Croen LA (2009). "Investigation of shifts in Autism reporting in the California Department of Developmental Services". *J Autism Dev Disord. May 29.*

Chapter XI

INDUSTRY

Knowing is not enough; we must apply. Willing is not enough; we must do. –
Johann Wolfgang von Goethe

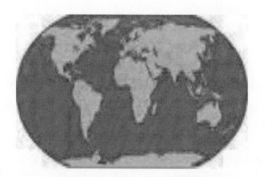

On Dain's 18th birthday, there were very few friends and relatives that gathered to celebrate and recognize his entry into adulthood. Allergy induced Autism had effected autistic behaviors to such an extent that it was difficult for others to be around him. Anguishing screams, biting his hands hard enough to draw blood, and hitting the top of his head with great force were cues that people meant uncertainty and frustration. Furthermore, darkened lower eyelids and blood shot eyes gave indications that his adaptive immune system continued to plague his health. Regressive Autism had severely altered his cognitive development over the last 18 years and medical science was helpless to intervene and reduce the progression of his allergy induced Autism. Because Dain lacked the basic skills to survive independently, constant care is required. Forever locked in a world of neurological dysfunction and in constant need of stimuli, Dain's parents would eventually make the decision to place him in an assisted living home for severely mentally disabled adults. Today the parents rejoice in his independence but helplessly lament his permanent mental and physical imprisonment.

WILL WE CONDUCT BUSINESS ETHICALLY AND PROFITABLY, AND EXERCISE LEADERSHIP AS RESPONSIBLE CORPORATE CITIZENS?

In the adhesive industry, there is an environmental standard initiative to supply "Green" adhesives having reduced hazardous ingredients. The term "Green" is often associated with natural-latex in that it is natural and substantially-free of volatile organic chemicals when extracted from the para rubber tree.

Will Corporate Citizenship in such Industries Affect the Health and Safety Issues associated with Natural-Latex?

In the spirit of Consumer health & safety, industrial organizations that sell natural-latex products were provided natural-latex allergy and allergy induced Autism information. The organizations were also presented information intended to better educate their customers about natural-latex allergy and initiate effective natural-latex exclusionary practices for children and adults.

As an example, in 2007 a letter was sent to a Fortune-500 Adhesive Company that sells natural-latex. The company website states that natural-latex adhesive applications include graphics arts, engineered systems, packaging, and converting.

The Adhesive Company responded to the letter as follows,

"There is not a compelling reason to pursue at this point in time."

Furthermore, in 2009 the same Adhesive Company was presented information on "Latex-Safe" Ultra low-protein natural-latex adhesives available from Vystar Corporation [1].

The Adhesive Company stated,

"We are not interested in Ultra low-protein natural-latex adhesives."

Is the Etiology of Allergy Induced Autism Created by Nature, Procreated by Immunity, Perpetuated by Science, and Maintained by Industry?

In some industries, only Government mandates will assure that "Latex-Safe" Ultra low-protein natural-latex will be used. Kudos to companies that recognize and act upon the health hazards associated with such allergenic proteins. An example is the H.B.Fuller Company; they presented a technical paper entitled, Replacing Natural Latex in Medical Device Packaging, presented at the Medical Packaging Symposium, January 17-19, 2000, Anaheim California. In addition their Company 'Vision Statement' is as follows, *"We are committed to the balanced interests of our customers, employees, shareholders and communities. We will conduct business ethically and profitably, and exercise leadership as a responsible corporate citizen."*

Corporate Citizenship and Government Mandates will be needed to help reduce natural-latex allergy. It is time to take responsibility for exposing atopic children to such allergens and start reducing exposure to future generations in that natural-latex allergy is preventable.

Where are the children we more often see
locked and entrapped neurologically:
our cries and our calls;
our attempts and our fear;
bring little to save what regresses each year;
slowly yet quickly the behavior takes seed;
a blossom rooted in disability;
everything changes;
dreams disappear;
what will come next is the maker of tears;
a child born with promise, a life turned complex;

unwanted stares and unending stress;
lost hope for the future brings;
what will come next...
Where are the children we more often see
locked and entrapped neurologically.

REFERENCES

[1]   Vytex™ Natural Rubber Latex website, http://www.vytex.com/

Chapter XII

SPIRITUALITY

Spirituality is the stone in stone soup; proper immunity is what the mind and body needs, then the stone can be enjoyed or discarded. – Michael J. Dochniak

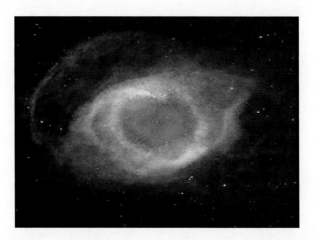

The Helix Nebula, sometimes called the "Eye of God"

At a very young age Dain was baptized in the Christian tradition wherein a trickle of holy water was sprinkled over his head and heartfelt prayers were spoken. A large gathering of worshipers witnessed the baptism and collectively all were pleased that this child was a member of the congregation and spirituality would be part of his life journey.

Spirituality has long been associated with religion, deities, the supernatural, and an afterlife. If spirituality is defined as the search for "God" within oneself, it is possible that the atypicality within Classical/Regressive Autism may affect ones ability to have a *sense of connection* and understand the meaning or potential existence of "God". Therefore, the state of awe, reverence, and wonder associated with spirituality may be lost.

Science is teaching us that the immune system is, and will continue to be, the architect that helps design our intellectual abilities. With a deeper knowledge of adaptive immunity, science has the ability to guide protein insult and affect the evolution of neuro-cognitive development in mankind; allowing everyone to pursue their spiritual quest.

RESOURCES

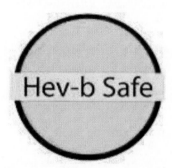

The following organizations, literature, or websites may be useful resources in finding out more information on natural-latex allergy.

American Latex Allergy Association
P.O. Box 198
Slinger WI 53086
1-888-972-5378
alert@latexallergyresources.org

The American Latex Allergy Association is a national non-profit 501, (c) (3), tax exempt organization that provides educational information about latex allergy and supports latex-allergic individuals. Originally, the organization was formed by a group of approximately 30 health care workers who acquired latex allergy. They provide information and support for one another, as well as to other persons and organizations. Their original name A.L.E.R.T., Inc. continues to reflect their mission: Allergy to Latex Education and Resource Team.

American Academy of Pediatrics
141 Northwest Point Boulevard
Elk Grove Village, IL 60007-1098
http://www.aap.org/

The American Academy of Pediatrics is an organization of 60,000 pediatricians committed to the attainment of optimal physical, mental, and social health and well-being for all infants and children.

A Book on Latex Allergy - Jordan N. Fink, MD. (1995). Latex Allergy. An issue of the series *Immunology and Allergy Clinics of North America*. W.B. Saunders Publisher.

Latex Allergy Law Website - http://www.megalaw.com/top/latex.php

United States Food and Drug Administration Website -
http://google2.fda.gov/search?q=latex+allergy&client=FDA&site=FDA&lr=
&proxystylesheet=FDA&output=xml_no_dtd&getfields=*&x=13&y=14

Natural Rubber Latex (NRL) Allergy Discussion Group http://www.immune.com/rubber/index.html

GLOSSARY

Adaptive Immunity	Highly specialized, systemic cells and processes that eliminate or prevent pathogenic challenges.
Adhesives	Polymeric material used for bonding substrates.
Allergy	Hypersensitive reaction to a substance harmless to most people.
Amino acids	A group of nitrogen-containing chemical compounds that form the basic structural units of proteins.
Androgen	Hormones that stimulate male characteristics.
Antibody	Proteins manufactures by the body and that bind to an antigen to neutralize, inhibit, or destroy it.
Antigen	any substance that, when introduced into the body, causes the formation of antibodies against it.
ASTM	Abbreviation for American Society for Testing and Materials
Atopy	A predisposition to various allergic conditions including eczema and asthma.
Autoimmune	A process in which antibodies develop against the body's own tissue.
Basophil	A type of white blood cell that is involved in allergic reactions.

B-cell	The principal functions of B cells are to make antibodies against antigens.
Blood-brain barrier	A special barrier that prevents the passage of materials from the blood to the brain.
Bromelain	The protein-digesting enzyme found in pineapple.
Candida albicans	A yeast common to the intestinal tract.
Carbohydrate	Sugars and starches.
Chronic	Long-term or frequently recurring.
Comorbidity	The effect of all other diseases or disorders that an individual might have other than the primary disease or disorder of interest.
Cross-reactivity	The reaction between an antigen and an antibody that was generated against a different but similar antigen.
Dementia	Senility. Loss of mental function.
Disaccharide	A sugar composed of two monosaccharides.
Endogenous Protein	A protein coming from inside the body.
Enzyme	An organic catalyst that speeds chemical reactions.
Epigenetics	Changes in phenotype (appearance) or gene expression caused by mechanisms other than changes in the underlying DNA sequence.
Estrogens	Hormones that produce female characteristics.
Etiology	The study of causation.
Exogenous Protein	A protein coming from outside the body.
Glucose	A monosaccharide that is found in the blood and is one of the body's primary energy sources.
Gluten	One of the proteins in wheat and certain other grains that gives dough its tough, elastic characteristic.
Guayule	Rubber obtained from the shrub of Parthenium argentatum.
Helper T-cell	Lymphocytes that help in the immune response.
Hevea brasiliensis	Natural-latex from the Para rubber tree

Hormone   A secretion of an endocrine gland that controls and regulates body function.

Iatrogenic   Meaning literally "physician produced", the term can be applied to any medical condition, disease, or other adverse occurrence that results from medical treatment.

Immunoglobulin-E   A class of antibody (or immunoglobulin "isotype") that has only been found in mammals.

Immunoglobulins   Antibodies

Innate Immunity   The cells and mechanisms that defend the host from infection by other organisms.

Incidence   The number of new cases of a disease or disorder that occurs during a given period (usually years) in a defined population.

In vitro   Outside a living body and in an artificial environment.

In vivo   In the living body of a person.

Latex   An aqueous colloid/emulsion of rubber particles.

LD50   The dose that will kill 50 percent of the animals taking the substance.

Leukocyte   White blood cell.

Leukotrienes   Inflammatory compounds produced when oxygen interacts with polyunsaturated fatty acids.

Mast cell   A cell, found in many tissues of the body, that contributes greatly to allergic and inflammatory processes by secreting histamine and other inflammatory particles.

Metalloenzymes   An enzyme that contains a metal at its active center.

Microflora   The microbial inhabitants of a particular region, e.g., colon.

Morphology   The study of the form or shape of an organism or part thereof.

Natural-Latex	The United States Food and Drug Administration terminology for natural rubber latex. Rubber obtained from botanical sources.
Neonate	A human infant less than a month old.
Synaptic Pruning	A synonym often used to describe the maturation of behavior and cognitive intelligence in children by "weeding out" the weaker synapses.
Neurotransmitters	Substances that modify or transmit nerve impulses.
Neurotrophins	A family of proteins that induce the survival, development, and function of neurons.
OSHA	Abbreviation for the Occupational Safety and Health Administration, US Department of Labor.
Papain	A protein-digesting enzyme of papaya.
Para Rubber	Hevea rubber from uncultivated trees.
Prenatal	The process in which an embryo or fetus (or *foetus*) gestates during pregnancy, from fertilization until birth.
Prevalence	The total number of cases of a disease or disorder in the population at a given time.
Polysaccharide	A molecule composed of many sugar molecules linked together.
Prostaglandin	Hormone-like compounds manufactured from essential fatty acids.
Protease	An enzyme that begins protein catabolism by hydrolysis of the peptide bonds that link amino acids together in the polypeptide chain.
T-cell	A lymphocyte under the control of the thymus gland.

INDEX

B

C

F

N

Q

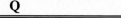

R